9.76

A GUIDE TO
GENERAL PRACTICE

GW00703526

A GUIDE TO GENERAL PRACTICE

THE OXFORD GP GROUP

Edited by Simon Street
and Andrew Wilkinson

SECOND EDITION

Blackwell Scientific Publications

OXFORD LONDON EDINBURGH
BOSTON PALO ALTO MELBOURNE

© 1979, 1987 by
Blackwell Scientific Publications
Editorial offices:
Osney Mead, Oxford, OX2 0EL
8 John Street, London, WC1N 2ES
23 Ainslie Place, Edinburgh, EH3 6AJ
52 Beacon Street, Boston
    Massachusetts 02108, USA
667 Lytton Avenue, Palo Alto
    California 94301, USA
107 Barry Street, Carlton
    Victoria 3053, Australia

First published 1979, Reprinted 1981 (twice)
Second edition 1987

DISTRIBUTORS

USA
    Year Book Medical Publishers
    35 East Wacker Drive
    Chicago, Illinois 60601

Canada
    The C.V. Mosby Company
    5240 Finch Avenue East
    Scarborough, Ontario

Australia
    Blackwell Scientific Publications
        (Australia) Pty Ltd
    107 Barry Street
    Carlton, Victoria 3053

British Library
Cataloguing in Publication Data

A Guide to general practice.— 2nd ed.
    1. Family medicine—Great Britain
    I. Oxford GP Group
    362.1′72′0941   R729.5.G4

    ISBN 0−632−01526−8

Photoset by Enset (Photosetting),
Midsomer Norton, Bath, Avon

Printed in Great Britain by
Butler & Tanner Ltd, Frome and London

Contents

Foreword

To have ten doctors newly trained in their vocation produce a *Guide to General Practice* is an exciting event. Here are clearly perceived needs met by a joint effort whilst still in training. Here is courage to help constructively those in the same position. Here is a demonstration of realistic self help.

This collection of data for every day represents an essential minimum for the doctor in his first plunge into General Practice. It gives information often buried in the experience of their elders or in books and circulars.

Such a guide should be a useful cornerstone on which to build. It should be followed by many editions as experience gained by the contributors is strengthened by increasing confidence.

These ten authors in training have set a high example that bodes well for the future of General Practice.

E. V. Kuenssberg
President of the Royal College of
General Practitioners

Preface to
First Edition

This handbook was written by general practice trainees during their training year. It is intended for trainees but should be of value to locums, assistants and new partners. It is a guide to the management of problems commonly encountered by doctors new to general practice. Details of medical treatment have been avoided deliberately. The material was selected from our experiences during the year. We were assisted by our trainers and other doctors to whom we are most grateful. We are also grateful to Jackie Sumner for her secretarial work.

Martyn Agass
Jeremy Bray
Robert Cave
Gillian Dean
Shirley Elliott

Richard Lloyd
Michael McGhee
Simon Street
Keith Sumner
Andrew Wilkinson

August 1978

Preface to Second Edition

The *Guide* has proved to be of value to trainees, locums, assistants and partners, new and established over the last eight years. This revision includes contributions from the original authors and also draws on the experience and comments of doctors and health professionals too numerous to list and thank.

Simon Street
Andrew Wilkinson
September 1986

The black bag

BLACK BAG — DIAGNOSTIC

Adhesive plasters
Clinical thermometer
Fluoresceine sticks
Foetal stethoscope
Gloves, jelly and tissues
Low reading thermometer
Needles
Ophthalmoscope
Otoscope
Patella hammer
Sphygmomanometer
Stethoscope
Swabs and specimen containers and transport medium
Syringes
Tape measure
Tongue depressors
Torch
Tourniquet
Tuning fork
Urine and blood dip sticks
Vaginal speculum

BLACK BAG – THERAPEUTIC

Injectable drugs
Adrenaline
Antiarrhythmics
Antibiotic
Anticonvulsant
Antiemetic
Antihistamine
Bronchodilator
Corticosteroid
Diuretic
Ergometrine
Glucagon or IV Dextrose
Major and minor tranquilliser
Opiate analgesic
Opiate antagonist

Oral drugs
Antacid
Antibiotics
Antidiarrhoeal
Antihistamine
Antipyretic
Bronchodilator
Corticosteroid
Diuretic
Major and minor analgesic
Sedative
Sugar lumps

Miscellaneous
Bronchodilator for nebuliser
Eyedrops
Glycerol suppositories
Ipecaccuanha
Paediatric antibiotics
Trinitrin

Drugs given from bag should be in a suitable container—glass or plastic, labelled with the following:

Patient's name
Drug name, dosage and quantity
Instructions, warnings and precautions
Name and address of Doctor
Date

BLACK BAG – ADMINISTRATIVE

Coins for telephone
Continuation cards
Controlled drugs record book
Dispensing forms
Emergency Treatment forms
Envelopes
Headed notepaper
Immediate Necessary Treatment forms
List of Chemists to dispense 'Urgent' prescriptions
Map
National Insurance Certificates
Obstetric calculator
Pathology forms
Prescription pad
Private certificates
Registration forms
Telephone numbers list
Temporary Resident forms
Therapeutic handbook

BLACK BAG – OPTIONAL EQUIPMENT

Airway
Antiseptic concentrate
Bandage and dressings
Drainage bag
ECG defibrilator
Epistaxis balloon
Giving set and fluids
IV Cannula
Nebuliser
Peak flow meter
Proctoscope
Scissors
Sterile dressing pack
Steristrips
Suturing equipment
Urinary catheters and spigots

BLACK BAG – OBSTETRIC

Equipment

Adult and neonatal
  endotracheal tube
Apron
Artery forceps
Calibrated jug
Dissecting forceps
Endotracheal tube
Episiotomy scissors
Giving set and fluids
IV cannula
Gloves
Laryngoscope
Light source
Mucus extractor

Needle holder
Neonatal laryngoscope
Obstetric cream
Obstetric forceps
Perineal retractor
Pudendal block needle
Sample bottles
Space blanket
Sterile dressing sheets
Suturing equipment
Swabs
Syringes and needles
Umbilical clamps
Urinary catheter

Drugs

Antibiotic
Concentrated antiseptic
Diazepam
Ergometrine
Hydrallazine

Local anaesthetic
Pethidine
Syntometrine
Vitamin K_1
Opiate antagonist

BLACK BAG – ROAD TRAFFIC ACCIDENT

Minimal equipment
Airway
Field dressings
Fire extinguisher
Fluorescent jacket
Giving set and fluid
IV cannula
Reflective warning triangle
Torch
Triangular bandages

Additional equipment
Blankets
Camera (with flash)
Cardiac monitor and defibrillator
Chest drain
Cut-down and surgical set
Dictaphone or notebook
Drugs for resuscitation
Endotracheal tubes
Entonox
Equipment for manual ventilation
Equipment for examination and blood samples
First aid kit including field and burns dressings
Flutter valve
Inflatable splints
Laryngoscope
Oxygen
Protective and identifying clothing
Radio telephone
Sucker
Suturing equipment
Warning signs and flashing beacon for car

BLACK BAG – DISPENSING

Carry prepacked containers of standard amounts, labelled
except for name and date dispensed.
Mark expiry date.
Mark filling level on bottles of dry powder for medicines.
Arrange collection/delivery of drugs not available from bag.
Special arrangements for drugs needing storage—vaccines,
insulin.

Analgesic—mild
       —moderate
       —opioid
Antacid
Antibiotic—broad spectrum
       —metranidazole
       —penicillinase resistant
Anticoagulant
Anticonvulsant
Antidepressant
Antidiarrhoeal
Antiemetic
Antihistamine
Antiparkinsonian drug
Antispasmodic
Antipsychotic/major tranquilizers
Benzodiazepine
β blocker
Bronchodilator
Digoxin
Diuretic—K^+ supplement
      —mild
      —strong
Ear/eye preparations—antibiotic
            —steroid

BLACK BAG — DISPENSING — continued

GTN
H_2 antagonist
Hypotensive
Inhalers—steroid
      —bronchodilator
Iron preparation
Laxative
Migraine preparation
NSAID
Oral contraceptives
Oral hypoglycaemic
Paediatric—antibiotic
      —antiemetic
      —antihistamine/sedative
      —electrolyte sachets
Skin—steroid
   —fungicide
Steroid

Medical practice

DESIRABLE WEIGHT CHART

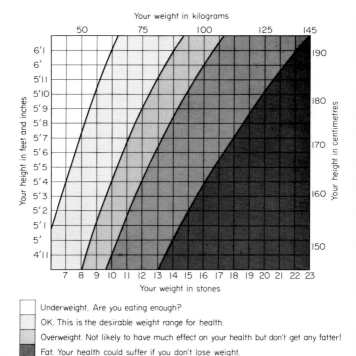

Your weight in kilograms

Your height in feet and inches

Your height in centimetres

Your weight in stones

Underweight. Are you eating enough?

OK. This is the desirable weight range for health.

Overweight. Not likely to have much effect on your health but don't get any fatter!

Fat. Your health could suffer if you don't lose weight.

Very fat. This is severe and treatment is urgently required.

Reproduced with the permission of Churchill Livingstone from *Treat Obesity seriously* by J. S. Garrow (1981).

DERMATOME CHART

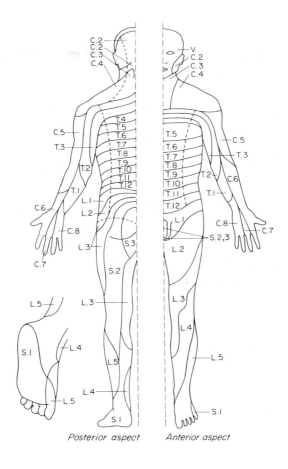

Posterior aspect   *Anterior aspect*

Reproduced with the permission of the Oxford University Press from *Brain's Clinical Neurology*, edited by R. Bannister (1978).

9

NORMAL VALUES OF PEAK EXPIRATORY FLOW—ADULT

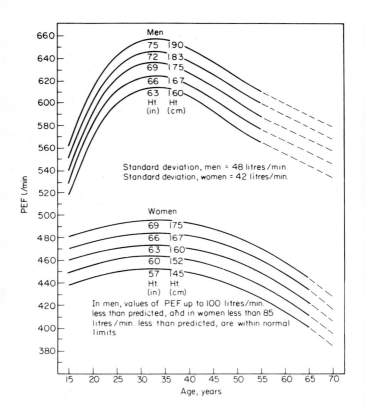

Courtesy of Clement Clarke International Ltd, Wigmore Street, London W1H 9LA

NORMAL VALUES OF PEAK EXPIRATORY FLOW–CHILDREN

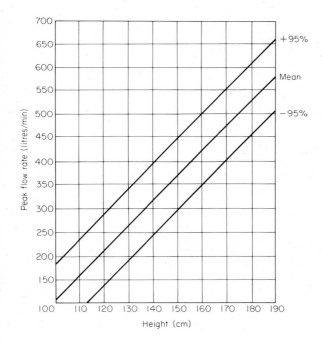

Normogram redrawn from original data of Godfrey *et al. British Journal of Diseases of the Chest*, **64**, 15 (1970). Reproduced by permission of Clement Clarke International Ltd, Wigmore Street, London W1H 9LA

11

FAMILY PLANNING

General advice

Methods of contraception
General knowledge of sex and sex function
Previous contraception
Discussion of reliability, convenience and disadvantages of the different methods with regard to age, parity, consort, and social factors
Instruction on use of contraceptives

Gynaecological history
LMP
Menarche
Menstrual cycle – frequency and complications
Past obstetric history
History of pelvic infection, abdominal or pelvic pathology
Rubella status

Examination
Weight and BP
General examination, including psychological—as indicated
Breasts
Pelvic examination
Cervical cytology
Urine analysis

Documentation
FP1001—Registration
FP1002—IUCD
FP1003—Temporary Resident

FAMILY PLANNING

The combined pill

Absolute contraindications
Thromboembolism
Severe Hypertension
Impaired Liver function
Oestrogen dependent tumours
Splenectomy
Otosclerosis
Pituitary disorder
Porphyria

Relative contraindications
More than 35 years
More than 10 years 'on the Pill'
Hypertension
Smoking
Family History of IHD
Diabetes
Depression
Migraine
Epilepsy
Renal disease
Valvular heart disease
Varicose Veins
Oligomenorrhoea
Breast Feeding
Contact Lenses

Side-effects

	Progestogen	Oestrogen
Too much	Depression	Hypertension
	Loss of libido	Recurrent migraine
	Ammenorrhoea	Premenstrual tension
	Breast discomfort	Breast discomfort
	Acne	Nausea and bloating
		Vaginal discharge
	Steady weight gain	Weight gain
	Recurrent thrush	
Too little	Breakthrough bleeding	Breakthrough bleeding
	Menorrhagia	

Follow up
Initially 3 months

Every 6 months
Every 3 years
Weight, BP
symptom review
As above
As above plus
pelvic examination
breast examination
cervical cytology

13

FAMILY PLANNING

Prostogen only pill

Absolute contraindications
Thromboembolism
Severe hypertension
Impaired liver function
Splenectomy
Otosclerosis
Porphyria

Relative contraindications
Smoking
Family history of IHD
Obesity
Diabetes
Contact lenses
Depression
Epilepsy
Renal disease
Valvular heart disease
Varicose Veins
Oligomenorrhoea

Side-effects
Too much
    Depression
    Loss of libido
    Ammennorrhoea
    Breast discomfort
    Acne
    Hirsuitism
    Steady weight gain
    Recurrent thrush
Too little
    Breakthrough bleeding
    Mennorrhagia

Follow up
Initially 3 months :
    Weight, blood pressure
    Symptom review

Every 6 months :
    As above
Every 3 years :
    As above plus—
    Pelvic examination
    Breast examination
    Cervical cytology

FAMILY PLANNING

Intra-uterine contraceptive devices

Medical history
LMP—for timing of insertion
Regularity of menses
Active infection
History of:
    Pelvic infection
    Heart valve diseases
    Anticoagulants and bleeding diatheses
    Anaemia
    Uterine malformation

Side effects
Increase in menstrual flow
Expulsion of IUCD
Lost threads
Pregnancy and ectopic pregnancy
Perforation
Infection and subsequent infertility
Pain

Follow up
After first period then annually
    Self examination
    Pelvic examination
    Side effects
    Change of IUCD – as indicated

FAMILY PLANNING

Rhythm methods
Temperature chart
Regular cycle
   'Unsafe Days' are Day 14 ± 4
Irregular cycle
   If the shortest cycle is x days and the longest cycle is y days
   then the 'safe' days are between $y-11$ and $x-18$
   Billings—Cervical mucus changes with ovulation

Barrier methods

Condom
With or without spermicidal creams or pessaries
No medical advice required

Diaphragm
Assess vaginal size and position of cervix
Follow up at 6 weeks and 6 months
Change cap every year

Traditional methods
Including coitus interruptus

Sterilisation
Counselling
Gynaecological or medical history
Reason for request
Stability of relationship
Attitude to parenthood
Examination
Technique of procedure
Permanence and reversibility
Low incidence of side effects or failure

FAMILY PLANNING

Post coital contraception

Oral

Two doses of combined oral contraceptive pill at 12 hr intervals to be started not later than 72 hours after intercourse

Typically 50 mcg Ethinyloestadiol/levonorgestrel

Two tablets repeated after 12 hours

Side effects

Nausea and vomiting

Increased tubal pregnancy rate

Check that menstruation occurs within 3 weeks

IUCD

Insertion not later than 72 hours after intercourse is another effective method.

FIRST ANTENATAL VISIT

History of present pregnancy
LMP, EDD, cycle, contraception, especially OC pill

Previous obstetric history
Pregnancy, labour, puerperium
Infant (alive or stillborn), weight, sex, gestation, neonatal
    problems
Feeding

Previous gynaecological history
Abortions – spontaneous or induced
Subfertility – investigations and treatment
Pelvic and abdominal surgery

General medical history
Hypertension and cardiac disease
Tuberculosis
Diabetes
Urinary tract infection, renal disease
Varicose veins
Psychiatric history—previous postnatal depression

Family history
Twins
Congenital abnormalities
General medical

Social history
Marital status
Smoking
Alcohol
Accommodation

Drugs
Current therapy
Allergies
Transfusions

FIRST ANTENATAL VISIT – continued

Examination
Weight, height, shoe size
Teeth, mucous membranes
Varicose veins
Blood pressure, heart sounds
Breasts
Abdomen – fundal height
Pelvic examination, cervical smear

Investigation
Urine, for microscopy, glucose, protein culture
Hb, blood group, WR, Rh antibodies
Rubella antibodies
Hepatitis antibodies
HTVL III antibodies
Consider ultrasound scan

Discussion
Antenatal care, parenthood classes
Amnio-centesis and genetic counselling
Diet, smoking, alcohol, drugs, X rays
Sexual intercourse, relaxation exercises
Dental care
Delivery and feeding
Postnatal social support

Forms:
FP 24, FW 8 (booking)
DHSS payments, Mat Bl (26 weeks)

Referral letter
Include all significant findings from the above assessment

Medical practice

SUBSEQUENT ANTENATAL VISITS

Follow–up
Monthly until 28 weeks
Then fortnightly until 36 weeks
Then weekly until term

History
Estimated dates
Symptoms – bleeding, pain
Foetal movements

Examination
Weight, urine analysis, BP
Oedema
Fundal height – dates?
Lie and position
Presentation
Engagement
Foetal heart

Investigations

12 weeks	Hb, antibodies
16–19 weeks	Alpha Feto Protein
28 weeks	Hb, antibodies if Rh negative
34 weeks	Hb, antibodies if Rh negative, vaginal examination and pelvic assessment

ANTENATAL CLASSES

Mothers' health
Exercise and relaxation
Diet, smoking, alcohol and pills
Mothers' questions and anxieties
Social contacts for new mothers
Maternity benefits

Hospital visit

The delivery
First, second and third stages
Pain relief
Caesarians, forceps and episiotomy
The neonate

Parentcraft
Feeding
Clothing
Bathing
Playing
Toys and equipment
Fathers' role
Emotional demands

FINAL POSTNATAL VISIT

Delivery
Date of delivery
Mode
Sex
Birth weight
Antenatal, perinatal or postnatal complications

Infant
Mode of feeding
Weight gain

Mother
Anaemia – oral iron therapy
Breast care
Bowels
Micturition
Lochia
Menstruation
Depression

Examination
Weight and blood pressure
Anaemia
Breasts
Abdomen – size of uterus
Perineum – episiotomy
Vulva and vagina
Cervix
Bimanual examination of uterus
Urine
Cervical smear

Discussion
Contraception – if not already using a method
Mother – child bonding
Complete FP24 etc
Register infant in practice
Immunisation and child care

CHILD HEALTH CLINIC

These are usually run by health visitors with either Local Authority doctors or general practitioners.

They provide a meeting place for mothers to discuss all aspects of child health amongst themselves or with professionals.

The doctor's role varies, but he is usually available for referrals from the health visitor, and takes an active part in the immunisation and developmental screening.

Most local authorities have a planned screening programme which should be regarded as a minimum. In a typical programme a child is seen at 2 months, 8 months and 18 months.

SCHOOL CLINIC

Organised by the Specialist in Community Medicine and Child Health responsible for area school health services.

Each child should attend the clinic during his second term, with his mother, child health clinic notes and teacher's notes.

Assessment is made of emotional, intellectual, social and physical development.

Examination
Appearance, height and weight
Gait
Motor ability
Speech
Visual acuity, squints
Colour vision
Hearing, audiometry

Failure or low attainment may merit reassessment or referral to a specialist agency via the general practitioner.

Medical practice

CHILD ASSESSMENT

Six week check

Average baby at 6 weeks	Smiles Eyes fixate and follow past midline Quietens to sound Head level momentarily in ventral suspension
Examination	Posture prone and ventral Weight Head circumference Heart sounds and femoral pulses Genitalia and hips Eye movements and squint Palate and fontanelle
Referral	Dislocated hips Heart murmurs Cataracts Persistent primitive reflexes Abnormal tone

CHILD ASSESSMENT

Eight month check

Average baby at 8 months	Sits unsupported Thumb/finger grasp Feeds himself Responds to more than 4 sounds
Examination	Weight Head circumference Hearing Vision distant and squint Dexterity Posture and tone Heart, hips, genitalia
Referral	Heart murmurs Failure to achieve milestones Failure to thrive

Medical practice

CHILD ASSESSMENT

Eighteen month check

Average toddler at 18 months	Walks, runs, climbs a chair Three words apart from 'mama' and 'dada' Builds tower of 3 bricks Drinks from cup
Examination	General physical Height, weight, Head circumference Genitalia Heart sounds Ears Vision, squint
Referral	Failure to achieve milestones Non walking Primitive reflexes or tone

CHILD ASSESSMENT

Three year check

Average child at 3 years

Jumps down steps, stands on
  one leg, rides a trike
Good language development
Can draw a man, copy circle
Normal socialisation with
  adults and other children

Examination

Height weight
Head circumference
General physical
Vision and squint
Hearing and ears

Referral

Abnormalities of above

DENVER DEVELOPMENTAL
SCREENING TEST

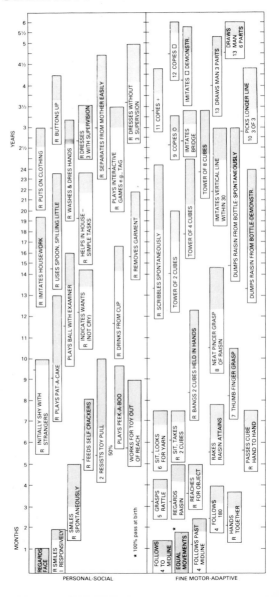

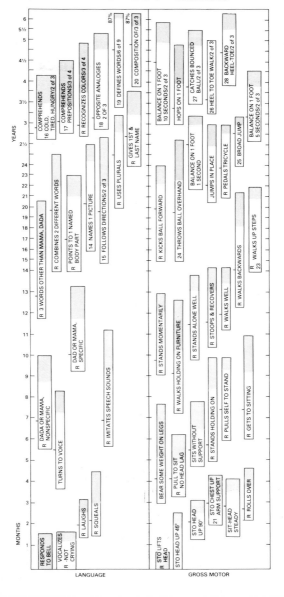

**DENVER DEVELOPMENTAL
SCREENING TEST—continued**

Directions
1. Try to get child to smile by smiling, talking or waving to him. Do not touch him.
2. When child is playing with toy, pull it away from him. Pass if he resists.
3. Child does not have to be able to tie shoes or button in the back.
4. Move yarn slowly in an arc from one side to the other, about 6'' above child's face. Pass if eyes follow 90° to midline. (Past midline; 180°.)
5. Pass if child grasps rattle when it is touched to the backs or tips of fingers.
6. Pass if child continues to look where yarn disappeared or tries to see where it went. Yarn should be dropped quickly from sight from tester's hand without arm movement.
7. Pass if child picks up raisin with any part of thumb and finger.
8. Pass if child picks up raisin with the ends of thumb and index finger using an overhand approach.
9. Get child to copy a circle. Pass any enclosed form. Fail continuous round motions.
10. Get child to indicate the longer of two lines (not bigger). Turn paper upside down and repeat. (3/3 or 5/6.)
11. Get child to copy a cross. Pass any crossing lines.
12. Get child to copy a square. Demonstrate if he fails. *When giving items, 9, 11 and 12, do not name the forms. Do not demonstrate 9 and 11.*
13. When scoring, each pair (2 arms, 2 legs, etc.) count as one part.
14. Get child to name animal picture. (No credit for sounds only.)
15. Tell child to: Give block to Mommie; put block on table; put block on floor. Pass 2 of 3. (Do not help child by pointing, moving head or eyes.)
16. Ask child: What do you do when you are cold? . . . hungry? . . . tired? Pass 2 of 3.

DENVER DEVELOPMENTAL SCREENING TEST—continued

Directions—continued

17. Tell child to: Put block *on* table; *under* table; *in front* of chair, *behind* chair. Pass 3 of 4. (Do not help child by pointing, moving head or eyes.)

18. Ask child: If fire is hot, ice is   ?; Mother is a woman, Dad is a   ?; a horse is big, a mouse is   ?. Pass 2 of 3.

19. Ask child: What is a ball? . . . lake? . . . desk? . . . house? . . . banana? . . . curtain? . . . ceiling? . . . hedge? . . . pavement? Pass if defined in terms of use, shape, what it is made of or general category (such as banana is fruit, not just yellow). Pass 6 of 9.

20. Ask child: What is a spoon made of? . . . a shoe made of? . . . a door made of? (No other objects may be substituted.) Pass 3 of 3.

21. When placed on stomach, child lifts chest off table with support of forearms and/or hands.

22. When child is on back, grasp his hands and pull him to sitting. Pass if head does not hang back.

23. Child may use wall or rail only, not person. May not crawl.

24. Child must throw overhand 3 feet to within arm's reach of tester.

25. Child must perform standing broad jump over width of test sheet. (8½ inches)

26. Tell child to walk forward, heel to toe, heel within 1 inch of toe. Tester may demonstrate. Child must walk 4 consecutive steps, 2 out of 3 trials.

27. Bounce ball to child who should stand 3 feet away from tester. Child must catch ball with hands, not arms, 2 out of 3 trials.

28. Tell child to walk backward, toe to heel, toe within 1 inch of heel. Tester may demonstrate. Child must walk 4 consecutive steps, 2 out of 3 trials.

Date and behavioural observations (how child feels at time of test, relations to tester, attention span, verbal behaviour, self-confidence, etc,):

31

BOYS' HEIGHT

Longitudinal standards for weight attained at given age. The shaded areas represent the 97th and 3rd centile limits of cross-sectionally derived standards.

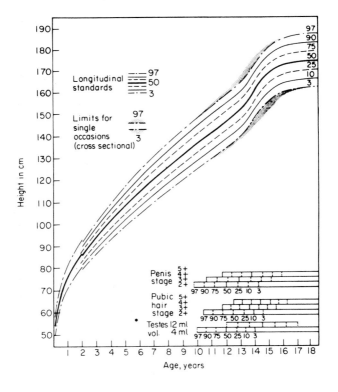

Prepared by Professor J.M. Tanner and Mr R.H. Whitehouse and reproduced by permission of Castlemead Publications, Hertford.

BOYS' WEIGHT

Longitudinal standards for weight attained at given age. The shaded areas represent the 97th and 3rd centile limits of cross-sectionally derived standards.

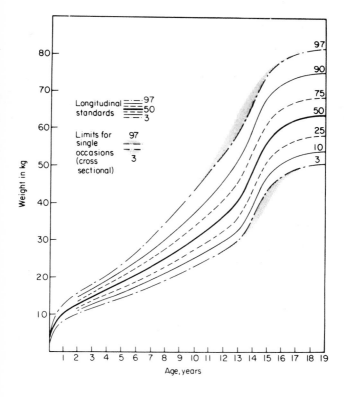

Prepared by Professor J.M. Tanner and Mr R.H. Whitehouse and reproduced by permission of Castlemead Publications, Hertford.

33

GIRLS' HEIGHT

Longitudinal standards for weight attained at given age. The shaded areas represent the 97th and 3rd centile limits of cross-sectionally derived standards.

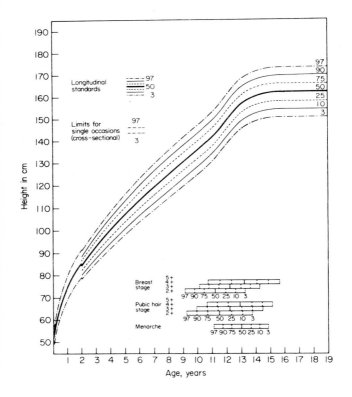

Prepared by Professor J.M. Tanner and Mr R.H. Whitehouse and reproduced by permission of Castlemead Publications, Hertford.

GIRLS' WEIGHT

Longitudinal standards for weight attained at given age. The shaded areas represent the 97th and 3rd centile limits of cross-sectionally derived standards.

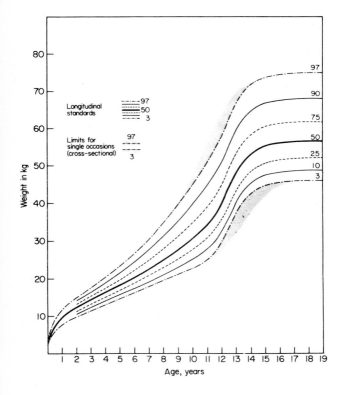

Prepared by Professor J.M. Tanner and Mr R.H. Whitehouse and reproduced by permission of Castlemead Publications, Hertford.

IMMUNISATION OF CHILDREN

History
General health
History of convulsions or cerebral irritability
Family history of convulsions
Strong reaction to previous injection
Allergy to eggs
Recent Febrile Illness
Steroids and immunosuppression

Procedure
Explanation of programme to mother
Consent
Intramuscular injections into deltoid or thigh
Three drops oral polio vaccine
Warn mother of possible reactions to immunisations

Documentation
Complete FP73 (including batch number)
Complete patient's personal vaccination card
Enter data and vaccination given in child's record card (FP7A)
Enter data on computer—if appropriate.
Complete Health Authority form

SUGGESTED IMMUNISATION PROGRAMME (see pp. 38–45 for notes)

Age	Vaccine	Dose & Route	Notes
3–6 mths.	Triple or Dip/Tet Polio (L*)	0.5 ml, IM 3 drops, oral	Interval between 1st & 2nd visits not less than 4 weeks
6–8 mths.	Triple (or Dip/Tet) Polio (L)	0.5 ml, IM 3 drops, oral	Interval between 2nd & 3rd visits not less than 4 weeks
9–14 mths.	Triple (or Dip/Tet) Polio (L)	0.5 ml, IM 3 drops, oral	
13–16 mths.	Measles (L)	0.5 ml, IM	
5 years	Dip/Tet Polio (L)	0.5 ml, IM 3 drops, oral	School entry
11–14 years	Rubella (L)	0.5 ml, SC	Girls only
13 years	BCG (L)	0.1 ml, intradermal	Tuberculin negative children only
15–19 years	Tetanus Polio (L)	0.5 ml, IM 3 drops, oral	School leavers

*Live vaccine

IMMUNISATION AGAINST DIPHTHERIA

Indications
Primary immunisation of all children under 10 years
Adults at risk of exposure with positive Schick test

Contraindications
Acute febrile illness
Aged more than 10 (if 25 Lf vaccine is used)

Side effects
Transient
    Fever
    Malaise
    Headaches
    Local reactions

Rarely
    Anaphylactic reactions
    Neurological reactions

Administration
0.5 ml by deep subcutaneous or intramuscular injection
25 LF Diphtheria toxin for children, 1.5 LF for adults.
Usually in combination with pertussis and/or tetanus
3 doses with intervals of 2 and 4 months starting at 3 months
    for children
3 doses with 1 month intervals for adults

IMMUNISATION AGAINST PERTUSSIS

Indications
All children from 3 months to 6 years, unless contraindicated

Contraindications
Acute febrile illness
History of reaction to a previous dose
History of cerebral irritation or damage as a neonate
History of fits or convulsions
Idiopathic epilepsy in parent or sibling
Development delays
Neurological disease

Side effects
Transient
  Fever
  Malaise
  Screaming
  Drowsiness
  Headache
  Local reactions

Neurological
  Febrile convulsion
  Encephalopathy
  Permanent brain damage

Administration
0.5 ml monovalent vaccine deep subcutaneous or intramuscular. Usually combined with diphtheria and tetanus
Three doses with intervals of 2 and 4 months. Start at 3
  months. Not indicated if child is more than 6 years

IMMUNISATION AGAINST TETANUS

Indications

Primary immunisation of children	(3, 6 and 9 months)
Post primary immunisation	(5 years)
Reinforcing dose for school leavers	(15–19 years)
Reinforcing dose for all adults	(every 10 years)
Special risk groups; farmers, gardeners	(every 5 years)
Primary immunisation for non-immune adults after sustaining open wounds	(as for children)

Contraindications
Acute febrile illness
Recent tetanus vaccination (less than 5 years)

Side effects
Local injection site reactions (up to 10 days)
Transient
    Headache
    Malaise
    Fever
    Lethargy
    Myalgia
    Urticaria

Anaphylactoid reaction (rare)
Peripheral neuropathy (rare)

Administration
Adsorbed tetanus toxoid (ATT)
0.5 ml vaccine by deep subcutaneous or intramuscular route.
Usually in combination with pertussis and/or diphtheria in children.
3 doses with intervals of 2 and 4 months

Human tetanus immunoglobulin (HTIG)

2.5 ml intramuscular	Available in hospital only
Indications	Delay in treating susceptible wound
	Devitalised tissue in wounds
	Puncture wounds
	Evidence of sepsis
	Immunosuppressed patients

IMMUNISATION AGAINST POLIO

Indications
Primary immunisation of all children	(3 months)
Post-primary immunisation	(5 years)
Reinforcing dose for school leavers	(15–19 years)
Special risks as adults	(every 10 years)

    Travelling in endemic or epidemic areas
    Health care workers in contact with polio cases
    Non-immune adults and parents in contact with individuals
       receiving vaccine

Contraindications (live vaccine)
Acute febrile illness
Steroids, radiation therapy, immunosuppression
Malignancy affecting immunological mechanism
1st trimester of pregnancy
Penicillin allergy (for IPV only)

Administration
Oral polio vaccine (OPV)
3 drops orally as drops on sugar lump.
Usually simultaneously with other primary vaccine in children

Inactivated polio vaccine (IPV)
0.5 ml subcutaneous or intramuscular for those in whom live
vaccine is contraindicated

IMMUNISATION AGAINST MEASLES

Indications
All children in their 2nd year (irrespective of a possible history
of previous measles infection)
Especially children:
With condition affecting growth
In residential care
Starting in playgroup, etc.
Within 3 days of exposure for non-immune contacts
Not routinely indicated for adults

Contraindications (live vaccine)
Acute febrile illness
Steroids, radiotherapy, immunosuppression
Malignancy affecting immunological mechanisms
Pregnancy
Allergy to neomycin or polymyxin
Anaphylactoid reactions to egg protein
History or family history of convulsions (unless human
immunoglobulin is given simultaneously)

Side effects
Reactivation of TB
Subclinical measles infection
Transient fever and malaise (within 10 days)
Anaphylactoid reactions

(The risk of encephalitis and subacute sclerosing encephalitis
is considerably less than with the natural disease.)

Administration
0.5 ml freshly mixed vaccine by deep subcutaneous or
intramuscular route

IMMUNISATION AGAINST RUBELLA

Indications
All girls between 10 and 14 years (irrespective of a possible history of previous rubella infection)
Non-immune women of child-bearing age (provided they are not pregnant and are using reliable contraception)
All non-immune women working with children

Contraindications (live vaccine)
Pregnancy
Acute febrile illness
Steroids, radiotherapy, immunosuppression
Malignancy affecting immunological mechanisms
Allergy to Neomycin or Polymixin
Allergy to rabbit protein (for 'Condevax')

Side effects
Teratogenesis in pregnant women
Transient
    Fever, sore throat
    Lymphadenopathy rashes
    Arthralgia, peripheral neuropathy (rare)

Administration
0.5 ml of freshly mixed vaccine by deep subcutaneous or intramuscular route
Inform all adult women of their rubella status

IMMUNISATION AGAINST TUBERCULOSIS

Indications
Those with a negative tuberculin test who are:
    Contacts of confirmed cases
    Children from high risk communities
    All neonates from high risk communities
    All health workers
    School children between 10 and 14 years
    Students in higher education

Contraindications (live vaccine)
Acute febrile illness
Dermatitis at injection site
Positive tuberculin test
Pregnancy
Steroids, radiotherapy, immunosuppression
Malignancy affecting immunological mechanisms
Recent administration of other live vaccine (3 weeks)

Side effects
Local reaction including ulcers, abscesses, and lymphadenitis
Anaphylactoid reaction

Administration
Careful intradermal injection of 0.1 ml of BCG vaccine into
    the deltoid region, after carrying out a tuberculin test

IMMUNISATION AGAINST INFLUENZA

Indications
Chronic chest disease
Chronic heart disease
Chronic kidney disease
Diabetes
Immunosuppression

Institutionalised and elderly
Health workers with heavy exposure to influenza

Contraindications
Allergy to eggs, Polymixin and Neomycin
Pregnancy (unless special need)

Side effects
Local skin reaction
Minor flu-like illness
Urticaria (very rare)

Administration
Composition of vaccine is reviewed annually
Vaccine may be 'whole virus', 'split virus' or 'surface antigen'
    and contain 1, 2 or 3 viruses.
Intramuscular or deep subcutaneous injection

COMMON INFECTIOUS DISEASES

Disease	Usual incubation period (days)	Interval between onset of illness and appearance or rash (days)	Minimum period of isolation providing the patient appears well
Chicken pox	10–21	0–2	Seven days from appearance of rash; all the scabs need not have separated
Dysentery (Sonne)	1–7	–	Until 24 hours after cessation of diarrhoea
Infective jaundice	14–42	–	Until clinical recovery
Measles	7–21	3–5	Until clinical recovery
Mumps	12–28	–	Until disappearance of all swelling
Rubella	14–21	0–2	Until clinical recovery
Scarlet fever	2–5	1–2	Until clinical recovery
Whooping cough	5–14	–	Until completion of antibiotics

There is no routine exclusion of contacts of any of these infectious diseases.
Exclusion is at the discretion of the doctor, i.e. children are special risk.

IMMUNISATION FOR TRAVELLERS

Recommended immunisations

Years of immunity given by immunisations.

	Tetanus	Polio	Cholera	Typhoid	Yellow Fever	Typhus
N. Europe & USA	10	10				
S. Europe, Middle East N. Africa & Far East	10	10	½	3		
Central Africa, Central & S. America	10	10	½	3	10	1
Canada, New Zealand & Australia			½			

Malarial prophylaxis is needed before entering certain countries; continue for 6 weeks after returning. Consult the BNF or recommendations by the local DHA.

Gamma-globulin injection may be required if travelling to countries where hepatitis is a risk.

Recommendations vary. Advice can be obtained from DHA, Tropical Diseases Hospital, Embassies or International Relations Division, DHSS 01-407-5522, Ex. 6711

Documentation

Complete any international certificates. State batch no. of vaccines.

Complete FP73 in detail including destination and countries en route.

Enter details including Batch No. in patient's notes.

Check certificate is completed fully and signed by patient and yourself.

Medical practice

CONTRAINDICATION TO IMMUNISATION FOR TRAVELLERS

	Anthrax	Cholera	Hepatitis B	Yellow fever	Typhoid	Polio	Tetanus
Acute infection		●	●	●	●	●	●
Chronic illness		●			●		
Severe reaction to previous immunisation		●					●
Steroids				●		●	
Immunosuppression				●		●	
Radiation				●		●	
Malignancy in immune system				●		●	
Pregnancy				●	●	●	
Age less 12 months		●			●		
Age less 9 months		●		●	●		
Allergy to:							
Neomycin				●			
Polymixin				●			
Penicillin						●(IPV)	
Egg protein				●			
No contraindications	●						

IMMUNISATION PROGRAMME

Standard programme

Day	Vaccine	Notes
Day 1	Yellow fever	At yellow fever vaccination centre
	1st Cholera	
	1st Oral polio	
Day 2 or 3	1st Typhoid	
	1st Tetanus	
Day 9 or 10	2nd Cholera	
Day 29	2nd Typhoid	If previously immunised against cholera, typhoid, tetanus and polio the relevant 2nd may be omitted
	2nd Tetanus	
	2nd Oral polio	
	Gamma Globulin	Give as close to departure as practicable

Rapid programme

Day 1	Yellow fever	
Day 15	Typhoid and Cholera	
	Gamma Globulin	

Emergency programme

When departure is within 24–48 hours, and cannot be delayed. There is an increased risk of systemic disturbance and this programme should be avoided if possible.

Day 1	Yellow fever – in the arm
	Typhoid and cholera – in the buttocks
	Gamma Globulin – in opposite buttock

Note. The WHO no longer recommends routine Smallpox vaccination. A Doctor's certificate advising against vaccination may be needed for some countries.

IMPORTED DISEASES

History
Country visited
Time and duration of visit
Itinerary and method of travel
Adequacy of prophylactic immunisation
The nature of anti-malarial and other precautions taken
Any other contacts at risk
Illness among other members of the party

Suggested investigations
Full blood count and ESR
Microscopy of thick and thin blood films
Clotted blood for culture, Widal and V¡ agglutinins
Stool specimens for microscopy and culture
Mid-stream urine for microscopy, culture and sensitivity
Chest X-ray

IMPORTED DISEASES —continued

Appearance of imported diseases.

Period	Disease	Countries visited
< 10 days	Endemic Typhus	N. India, Pakistan, SE. Asia, Far East, Pacific, Queensland, Africa
	Dengue	Tropics, Sub-tropics,
	Yellow Fever	Africa, Central and South America
Up to 21 days	Malaria (perhaps longer)	Tropics and Sub-tropics
	Typhoid	Tropics, Sub-tropics, Mediterranean
	Trypanosomiasis	Africa 12°N−25°S
	Schistosomiasis	
	(a) haematobium	Nile, Africa, Iraq, Bombay, Mid and Far East
	(b) mansoni	Nile, Africa, Arabia, Central and South America
	Brucellosis	Worldwide
	Tropical Haemorrhagic Fever	West Africa
> 21 days	Kala-azar	North, East, West Africa, Central America, South America China, East India
	Viral Hepatitis	Worldwide
	Filariasis	Africa, SE. Asia, North Australia, West Indies, South America, Pacific
	Amoebiasis	Tropical and Sub-tropical

NOTIFIABLE DISEASES

The Health Service and Public Health Act 1968 requires a doctor to notify the local Community Physician (Environmental Health) if a person is suffering from one of the following infectious diseases:

Acute encephalitis
Acute meningitis
Acute poliomyelitis
Anthrax
Cholera
Diphtheria
Dysentery –
   amoebic or bacillary
Food poisoning –
   actual or suspected
Infective Jaundice
Lassa fever
Leprosy
Leptospirosis
Malaria
Marburg Disease

Measles
Ophthalmia neonatorum
Paratyphoid fever A or B
Plague
Rabies
Relapsing fever
Scarlet fever
Smallpox
Tetanus
Tuberculosis
Typhoid fever
Typhus fever
Viral haemorrhagic fever
Whooping cough
Yellow fever

Notification, for which a fee is paid, should be made on a certificate obtainable from the DHA or the local government District Environmental Health Department.

Scotland and Northern Ireland
Regulations vary from the above list.

INDUSTRIAL DISEASES

Notifiable diseases

These are a group of diseases which, when they occur in factories, are compulsorily notifiable by doctors and employers to the Health and Safety Executive.

Aniline poisoning
Anthrax
Arsenical poisoning
Beryllium poisoning
Cadmium poisoning
Carbon disulphide
  poisoning
Chrome ulceration
Chronic benzene
  poisoning

Compressed air sickness
Epitheliomatous
  ulceration
Lead poisoning
Manganese poisoning
Mercury poisoning
Phosphorus intoxication
Toxic anaemia
Toxic jaundice

If in doubt consult Employment Medical Advisory Service or local Health and Safety Executive.

'Prescribed' diseases

Compensation is payable under the National Insurance (Industrial Injury) Act 1946. The occupations responsible and the list of prescribed diseases are laid down in the Schedule of the Department of Health and Social Security.

USE OF LABORATORY

It is a DHSS recommendation that all GPs have access to hospital laboratories. Pathologists will provide a domiciliary service on request and will discuss any problems with the doctor.

Supplies
FPC
> Sterile disposable plastic syringes
> Needles

Laboratory
> Lists of normal values
> Lists of appropriate containers
> Request forms
> Suitable packaging
> containers, transport media, swabs

Specimens
Specimens and forms should be similarly labelled with:
> Patient's full name
> Date of birth
> Address
> GPs name and address
> Date and time specimen taken
> NHS or private patient

Full clinical information should be supplied:
> Date of onset
> Symptoms
> Diagnosis
> Relevant treatment
> Hepatitis or high risk warning on card and specimen

Transportation
There are usually arrangements with the local laboratory or alternatively specimens can be delivered by the patient or by first class mail. Post Office regulations demand that specimens be in a sealed receptacle in a strong Post Office approved box with sufficient material to prevent leakage if damaged, and marked 'Fragile – with care' and 'Pathological specimen'.

USE OF LABORATORY – Continued

Public Health Laboratory Service
It serves community physicians, general practitioners, and hospitals with responsibility directly to the Secretary of State for Health and Social Security.

Routine Work – comprehensive bacteriological service
Investigation – epidemiology, prevention and control of infectious disease
Advice – to central and local health authorities
Research

High risk groups
Known infectious disease carriers
Hepatitis A or B, syphilis, or AIDS
Chronic liver disease
Jaundice of unknown origin
Haemodialysis
Haemophilia
Immunosuppressive treatment
Organ transplantation
Drug addiction
Sexual contacts of high risk patients

Procedure
Discuss with laboratory
Doctor should take specimens
Plastic gloves and appropriate protective clothing
Screw-capped containers
Specimen and request form labelled in approved manner
Specimens placed in plastic bag, separate from forms

Disposal of needles and syringes
Make special arrangements with waste disposal authority or hospital for disposal of sharps and contaminated waste

Check lists

CONSULTATION TASKS

1 To define the reasons for the patient's attendance, including:
(i) the nature and history of the problems;
(ii) their aetiology;
(iii) the patient's ideas, concerns, and expectations;
(iv) the effects of the problems.
2 To consider other problems:
(i) continuing problems;
(ii) at risk factors.
3 To choose with the patient an appropriate action for each problem.
4 To achieve a shared understanding of the problems with the patient.
5 To involve the patient in the management and encourage him to accept appropriate responsibility.
6 To use time and resources appropriately.
7 To establish or maintain a relationship with the patient which helps to achieve the other tasks.

The above list is reproduced from *The Consultation* by D. Pendleton, T. Schofield, P. Tate and P. Havelock (1984), with the permission of Oxford University Press.

CONTINUING CARE
Case finding
Disease register	Entry criteria
	Screening or case finding
Call and recall system	Computer or manual

Cooperation
Patient compliance	Full discussion
	Shared clinical objectives
	Cooperation cards
	Regular follow up
Primary care colleagues	Administration and secretarial
	Nurse support Partners role
Consultant colleagues	Shared care and Supportive role Specialist advise Technical backing

Control
Passive/Monitoring	Patient; symptom charts, etc.,
	Doctor; regular recording of objective indicators
Active/Intervention	Patient; Titrate therapy against severity
	Doctor; initiate changes in objectives and management

Complications
Prevention	Advise on preventive measures
	Detect and intervene early with preventable complications
Mitigation	Monitor progress of any unavoidable complications
	Educate to avoid exacerbations

Continuity
	Recall regularly
	Review objectives
	Revise protocols
	Renew motivation and rewards
	Reinforce cooperation
	Audit

Check lists

PSYCHO-SEXUAL HISTORY

Present complaint

Personal history
Childhood and friends
Family inter-relationships
School and achievements
Religious and moral attitudes
Marital history
Extra-marital history

Sexual history
Sex education
Family attitudes and taboos
Traumatic experiences
Puberty
Masturbation
Homosexuality
First sexual experiences
Subsequent sexual experience
Present sexual relationship

Present sexual function
Libido
Arousal
Potency
Ejaculation
Orgasm
Frequency of intercourse
Variations

Past medical history

Past obstetric and gynaecological history

Past psychiatric history

Social history

Drugs

Examination

Investigations

PRE-CONCEPTION CHECK

DISCUSSION

Present family planning
Medical and obstetric history
Family history of both partners
Place of delivery
Role of midwife
Genetic counselling as appropriate, seek specialist advice
Smoking
Alcohol
Drugs e.g. anticonvulsants
    long-term antibiotics
    or immuno-suppressives

Investigation
Blood pressure
Urinalysis
Weight
Rubella titre – and vaccination
Full blood count
Blood group
Rhesus antibodies
Syphilis serology
Hb electrophoresis. Sickle cell and thalassaemia
Breast examination
Pelvic examination and smear

SPORTS INJURY

History
Sport
Action causing injury
Severity of injury
Loss of consciousness
Level of performance
Training schedule
Forthcoming fixtures
Protective equipment
Techniques
Previous injuries

Examination
Impairment of function
Bone injury
Soft tissue injury
Visceral injury

Aims of treatment
Appropriate first aid
Restoration of function
Preservation of fitness
Prevention of recurrence
Restoration of confidence

REHABILITATION

Definition
The restoration of patients to their fullest physical, mental and social capability

Areas to consider
Avoidable disability
Physical and mental health
Aids and appliances
Return to work
Community involvement
Self-help groups and support for careers
Sexual activity
Information and health education

Rehabilitation teams may comprise:

Doctors	Occupational Therapist
Health Visitor	Physiotheropist
Nurse	Remedial Gymnast
Social Worker	Speech Therapist
Disablement Resettlement Officer	

Role of GP
Early treatment of disease
Long term medical supervision
Co-ordination of help in the community
Support for patient, family and friends

Rehabilitation of coronary patient
Patient with uncomplicated myocardial infarction will normally be capable of normal range of physical activity, including sexual intercourse, within 4–6 weeks.

Important to avoid long term disability by encouraging activity

Some hospitals now have Coronary Rehabilitation Programmes

Certain occupations are affected by history of myocardial infarction e.g. PSV driver

ASSESSMENT OF THE DISABLED

Medical support
Drug therapy
Nursing care
Occupational therapy
Physiotherapy

Locomotion
Aids to daily living
Sticks, frames and wheelchairs
Tricycle, car and bus

Accommodation
Access
Doors and floors
Bathroom and toilets
Heating and cooking
Warden controlled flat
Part III accommodation

Social support
Food, shopping and laundry
Family and neighbours
Home help
Meals on wheels
Societies
Clubs and churches
Day care centres
Voluntary organisations
Financial help

ASSESSMENT OF THE ELDERLY

Risk factors
Extreme age
Chronic illness
Immobility
Loneliness
Recent bereavement
Poverty

Medical assessment
Weight, BP, urine
Teeth and dentures
Sight and hearing
Bowel and bladder function
Drug regimen
Assessment for dependency

Psychiatric assessment
Intellectual function
Orientation and memory
Psychiatric symptoms
Social crises

Accommodation
Access
Stairs and alterations
Heating and lighting
Bathroom and toilets
Housework and hygiene
Laundry and shopping
Cooking and diet
Part III accommodation

Social support
Family and neighbours
Health visitors and social workers
Bath attendant and chiropodist
Helping agencies, disease societies and self-help groups
Day care
Hospital arrangements
Finance, pensions and benefits

Check lists

FITNESS TO DRIVE

Patients over 70 require 3-yearly medical certificates.

The patient, holding or applying for a licence, is himself obliged to notify the Licensing Authority if he is suffering from a relevant or prospective disability.

The doctor should act as adviser to his patient. He should use his own discretion in informing the Licensing Authority if he thinks that the driving of a patient could be a danger. A medical defence society should be consulted if there is a potential breach of confidence.

History
Driving habits: local, rush hour, professional, experience
Coronary, heart disease, aortic valve disease
Diabetic hypoglycaemia
Epilepsy
Transient cerebral ischaemia, Ménières disease
Vertigo, Parkinsonism, multiple sclerosis
Limb disability
Severe deafness
Monocular vision, diplopia, night blindness
Subnormality, illiteracy, psychiatric breakdown
Dementia
Drugs

Examination
Heart rate, heart sounds, blood pressure
Power, co-ordination, sensation
Visual acuity, fields and fundi
Hearing

Investigation
Urine, ECG, if indicated

The doctor must refer to the current guidelines* on medical requirements for different licences.

*See Consulting Room Bookshelf, p. 159

TRAVEL BY AIR –
CONTRAINDICATIONS

Cardiovascular disease
Myocardial infarction (within 6 weeks of onset)
Uncompensated cardiac failure. Patients with angina or
    controlled cardiac failure may be carried but extra oxygen
    will be supplied
Recent cerebral infarction
Severe anaemia including sickling disorders

Respiratory tract
Severe otitis media or sinusitis, or recent middle ear surgery
    or eustachian catarrh
Pneumothorax
Irreversible airways disease
Within 21 days of major chest surgery

Gastrointestinal
Within 10 days of simple abdominal operation
Within 3 weeks of G.I. haemorrhage
Colostomies are acceptable if extra dressings are carried

Central nervous system
Epilepsy – acceptable if extra anti-convulsants are carried
Mental illness if without escort and sedation

Diabetes
Diabetic passengers may travel if they manage their own
    medication. Special diets provided. Note time zone change
    on arrival at destination

Infectious diseases

Pregnancy
Beyond 35 weeks gestation for international journeys and 36
    weeks gestation for short flights

Air in body cavities
Introduction of air to body cavities for diagnostic or
    therapeutic purposes within 7 days

Fractured mandible with wiring

Check lists

'THE MOT'

'The MOT' is a minimal health check designed to identify and reduce risk factors for heart disease and stroke. It is part of the extended role of the practice nurse usually assisted by a clinical 'facilitator'.

Identify the at-risk population   (35–65 years)

Call and recall system   (5 year intervals)
    (1 year if at risk)

Monitor and record
Blood pressure
Height
Weight
Ideal weight
Smoking habits
Oral contraceptive use
Family history (1st degree relatives with history of myocardial
    infarction, diabetes or stroke)

Case finding
Hypertension
Diabetes
Hypercholesterolaemia

Offer advice
Smoking
Diet
Exercise

Referral as appropriate

Opportunistic preventive care
Cervical cytology
Breast examination
Immunisations

ABBREVIATIONS

ACBS	Advisory Committee on Borderline Substances
AHCPA	Association of Health Centre and Practice Administrators
AMS	Association of Medical Secretaries
AMSPAR	Association of Medical Secretaries, Practice Administrators and Receptionists
BMA	British Medical Association
BNF	British National Formulary
CAB	Citizens' Advice Bureau
CHC	Community Health Council
CSM	Committee for the Safety of Medicines
DHA	District Health Authority
DHSS	Department of Health and Social Security
FPC	Family Practitioner Committee
GPFC	General Practice Finance Corporation
GMSC	General Medical Services Committee
HEC	Health Education Council
HVA	Health Visitors' Association
JCPTGP	Joint Committee on Postgraduate Training for General Practice
LMC	Local Medical Committee
MDU	Medical Defence Union
MIMS	Monthly Index of Medical Specialties
MPC	Medical Practices Committee
MPS	Medical Protection Society
MRC	Medical Research Council
MWF	Medical Womens Federation
NCC	National Consumer Council
NIC	National Insurance Contribution
OHE	Office of Health Economics
PPA	Prescription Pricing Authority
PPG	Patient Participation Group
RCGP	Royal College of General Practitioners
RCN	Royal College of Nursing
RHA	Regional Health Authority
RMO	Regional Medical Officer
SFA	Statement of Fees and Allowances ('The Red Book')
SSP	Statutory Sick Pay
WHO	World Health Organisation

STRUCTURE OF THE NHS

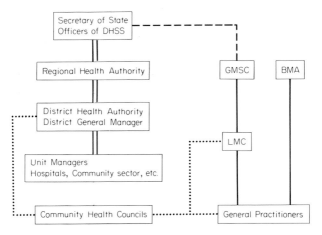

Key

(═══════) Accountable

(. . . . .) Co-opted representation

(─────────) Elected representation

(– – – – – –) Negotiates

STRUCTURE OF THE FPC

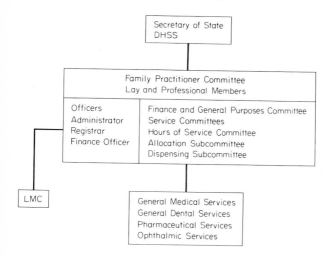

EDUCATIONAL COMMITTEES

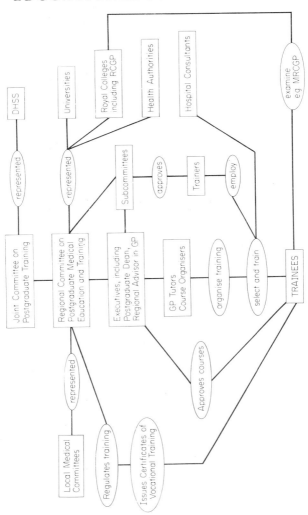

The detailed structure varies from region to region

MEDICO – POLITICAL COMMITTEES

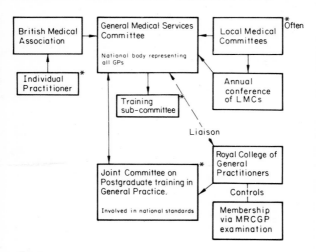

*Representation by GP trainees. There may be local variations.

THE REGIONAL MEDICAL SERVICE OF THE DHSS

The RMS acts as an independent referee when there is doubt about a patient's capacity for work. It is the regionally based branch of the DHSS Headquarter Medical Division responsible for primary care. It is divided into six divisions, based on Leeds, Nottingham, Manchester, Birmingham, Reading and Stanmore, with 40 Medical Officers working under the supervision of six Divisional Medical Officers who have considerable experience as principals in general practice.

References are made to the RMS by the Social Security side of the Department where incapacity appears unduly prolonged. After seeing reports from Doctors, RMOs can deal with about half these references without the need for examination, as long as the reports contain sufficient additional information.

An RMO tries to visit each practice in his area every two years to discuss matters of mutual interest relating to primary care and departmental policies. The meeting may cover such topics as NHS administration, the staffing of general practice, including medical, nursing and ancillary staff, practice organisation, practice premises, services to patients, hospital services, prescribing, the reference system, postgraduate education and new trends in practice. When an RMO makes an appointment to visit a practice, it is helpful if 30–40 minutes can be set aside for the appointment and if all the partners can arrange to be present.

The RMO also visits GPs to discuss high cost prescribing and self-audit prescribing analyses requested by GPs, to promote more effective prescribing. Two RMOs in each division specialise in practice premises, offering advice to GPs and FPCs about the Medical aspects, the Cost Rent Scheme and the provision of Improvement Grants.

Although an RMO is never involved in any formal proceedings, he may advise GPs about their obligation under certain Acts and Regulations, including the Misuse of Drugs Act, the terms of service and the regulations relating to the issue of doctors' statements for Social Security purposes.

ORGANISATION OF SOCIAL SERVICES

Social services Departments are run by local authorities and vary from area to area. A department will be divided by functions

Research, Development and Training

Personnel

Administration and Finance

Domiciliary Social Work. General Medical and Psychiatric Social Workers. Area Offices

Domiciliary Support Services. Home helps, Meals on Wheels, voluntary services

Care Services—residential and day care

Northern Ireland
Health & Social Services are integrated.

PATIENT PARTICIPATION GROUPS (PPG)

Patient participation groups are local and autonomous groups of patients. Their aim is to improve primary care by supporting their primary care team, to promote mutual trust, and to co-ordinate consumer activities:

Feedback on existing services
Accessibility
Acceptability
Responsiveness to need
Effectiveness

Feedback for planning new services

Complaints/grievances/suggestions

Health education
Specialist lectures
Education on health beliefs
Leaflets, posters, audiovisual aids
Use of media

Support of primary health care
Transport
Prescription collection

Self-help groups

Community care
Elderly
Young mothers
Disabled
Social events
Communications

Lobbying outside bodies
Health Authorities
Local Government
Central Government

74

HELPING AGENCIES

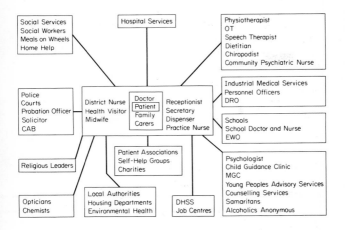

Check lists

REASONS FOR REFERRAL

Emergency care
Assessment and management

Diagnosis
Expert second opinions
Exclusion of suspected pathology

Investigation
Specialist knowledge (e.g. Immunopathology)
Technical facilities (e.g. X-rays)

Treatment
Technical skills and facilities
    (e.g. surgery, chemotherapy)
Specialist skills
    (e.g. psychiatry, dermatology)

Continuing care
Advice on symptom control
Assessment of complications

Doctor: patient relationship
New initiatives in 'difficult cases'
Patient's request for a second opinion

STANDARD REFERRAL LETTER

To be effective a letter to a consultant should be brief. It should include the detailed information that he may not be able to obtain from the patient himself.

Name, age, address
Marital status, occupation, hospital number

Reason for referral
Opinion or action requested
Degree of urgency

Time scale of events
Relevant personal and family history
Relevant findings on examination and investigation

Drug regimen
Drug idiosyncrasies
Patient compliance
Social factors
What the patient has been told
Future management

REFERRAL LETTERS — SPECIAL CASES

In certain circumstances special information will be of value to the hospital staff in addition to the standard referral letter.

Obstetric—see page 19.

Paediatric
Pregnancy and parental attitude to pregnancy
Neonatal and developmental history
History of family dynamics
History or suspicion of child abuse

Sterilisation or vasectomy
Origin of request
Doctor's opinion
Obstetric and gynaecological history
Contraceptive history
Stability of relationship

Termination of pregnancy
History of present pregnancy – LMP gestation
Obstetric and gynaecological history
Medical and psychiatric history
Reasons for request
Patient and family's attitude
Doctor's recommendation
Documentation

Overdose—see page 85

Psychiatric
Full details of present illness and associated disorders
Change in personality or intellect
Previous psychiatric illnesses
Past medical history
Drugs and alcohol
Personal and social history
Family psychiatric illness
Family background

78

EMERGENCY PSYCHIATRIC ADMISSIONS

Under the 1983 Mental Health Act, an application can be made for compulsory admission 'where the patient is suffering from a mental disorder warranting detention for their own health or safety or for the protection of others'.

Section 2
Compulsory admission for 28 days for 'assessment'
Application by next of kin or approved social worker
Recommendation by two doctors
Contact duty psychiatrist and social worker and arrange home visit

Section 3
Compulsory admission for 6 months for 'treatment'
Application by approved social worker or nearest relative
Recommendation by two doctors
Contact duty psychiatrist and social worker

Section 4
'Emergency' admission for 72 hours for assessment
Application by approved social worker or nearest relative
Recommendation by one doctor

Notes. The social worker is responsible for all documentation and the transport of the patient to hospital.

Scotland and Ireland
The Mental Health Act (Scotland) 1960 provides for compulsory admission under Section 24. The application is made by the nearest relative or mental welfare officer together with a medical recommendation, which must be approved by the Sheriff. In an emergency Section 31 allows the patient to be detained for 7 days.

Check lists

NON-ACCIDENTAL INJURIES TO CHILDREN

History
Declared anxiety of battering
Inappropriate, devious or changing story
Varying reports from different witnesses
Delay in seeking help
Previous unexplained injury
Identify risk factors
    Changes in doctors
    Repeated visits by an anxious mother with a child
    Separation from parents including neonatal period
    Parents subjected to battering
    Social circumstances
    Mental illness in parents
    No helping relatives or friends
    Unrealistic expectations of child
    Apathy or lack of concern for child

Examination
Bruises including petechiae, repetitive bruising, finger and thumb prints, bruises from adult bites
Fractures without a history of accident (radiological appearances include multiple fractures and various stages of healing)
Burns and scalds including cigarette burns
Mouth bruising and lacerations
Skull – fractures, subdural haematoma, retinal haemorrhages
Visceral injuries
General neglect

Action
Health visitor
Social worker
Community physician
Paediatric unit
Place of safety
Police as appropriate

PROBLEM FAMILIES

Persistent truancy
Juvenile delinquency
Probation Order
Care Order
Child Guidance Clinic
Prolonged separation from parents
Repeated hospital treatment
Repeated accidents

Size of family
Maternal age
Family history
Single parent – divorced or separation
Marital problems
Prolonged mental or physical illness
Employment
Finance and benefits
Alcohol, gambling, sex and violence
Criminal record
Suspected child abuse

Housing
Personal and domestic hygiene
Domestic mismanagement
Helping agencies

BODILY ASSAULT

This examination is best conducted by a police surgeon and will involve a written report and possible court appearance.

Procedure
Consent
Chaperone
Suitable premises and lighting
Detailed account of all findings
Photograph or drawing where appropriate
Claim appropriate fee and mileage

History
Date, time, place of incident
Course of events, persons involved, witnesses
Loss of consciousness
Previous medical history
Drugs
Alcohol

Examination
General appearance
Inspect clothing
General examination
Careful examination of any injuries
Age of bruising
Neurological examination

Investigations
X-rays where appropriate
The police will specify what samples are required for the forensic laboratory

SEXUAL ASSAULT

This examination is best conducted by a police surgeon and will involve a written report and possible court appearance.

Procedure
Written consent from victim, parents or guardian
Chaperone
Suitable premises and lighting
Change of clothing for victim
Establish that sexual intercourse has occurred
Detailed account of all findings
Claim appropriate fee and mileage

History
Date, time, place of incident
Course of events, persons involved, witnesses
Resistance by victim
Menstrual history

Examination
General appearance and behaviour
Apparent age
Inspect clothing
General examination
Nails
Genitalia
Pubic hair

Investigations
Venous blood
Swabs for semen
Clothing fragments
Foreign hairs
Dried blood
The police will specify what samples are required for the forensic laboratory

INTOXICATION WITH ALCOHOL

A doctor is usually only required to take a venous blood sample. The kit is provided by the police. Verbal consent should be obtained.

When examination is required, first obtain written consent.

History
Medical history
Psychiatric history
Previous personality
Medication
Drug abuse

Examination
General appearance and behaviour
Careful examination of any injuries
Mouth and breath
Pulse, blood pressure
Temperature
Skin
Ears and hearing
Eyes
Gait, co-ordination, stance
Mental state, memory
Writing ability

Investigations
Breath test
Urine
Blood for alcohol and drug levels
Blood sugar
Prepare written report and keep copy
Claim fee and mileage from police

OVERDOSE AND SELF INJURY

History
Date, time, place of incident
Course of events, persons involved, witnesses
Evidence of overdose
Quantity, type of drug or poison
Alcohol
Previous attempt
Previous medical history
Previous psychiatric history
Social factors

Examination
General appearance and behaviour
Level of consciousness
General examination
Careful examination of any injuries
Depression, hysteria, other psychiatric symptoms

Management
First aid care
Hospital admission
Retain any medicines or poisons for identification
Contact Poison Centre
Care of dependents
Follow up

Referral letter
Explicit circumstances and evidence of overdose
Any known psychiatric history
Known supportive persons

Check lists

ROAD TRAFFIC ACCIDENT

Procedure
Ensure personal safety
Wear reflective jacket
Park car to protect casualties, provide light and warn traffic
Assess number of casualties and continuing risk
Call emergency services
Find and sort casualties
Delegate care where possible
Avoid moving casualties
Co-operate with rescue services

First aid care
Airway and Respiration
Circulation
Stop massive haemorrhage
Pain relief
Stabilise fractures
Exclude spinal injury
Hypothermia
Record medical events and treatment given
Ensure hospital is informed

CORONER'S CASE

Death due to suspected unnatural cause
Cause of death uncertain
No medical attendance in previous fourteen days
Previous accident or injury
Allegations of negligence
Industrial disability or war pension
Alcoholism or self neglect
Death of infant or fostered child
Death due to drugs, poisons or medical treatment
Death due to abortion unless spontaneous
Death in custody or prison
Death in road traffic accident
Death due to factory accident
Suicide

The coroner will issue death certificate, request post-mortem and sign cremation forms.

Scotland
In Scotland the Procurator-Fiscal acts instead of the Coroner.

There is no compulsion to notify death in Scotland except in the case of fatal accidents and death in suspicious circumstances.

The public inquest in England has its counterpart in the Scottish precognition, which is conducted in private by the Procurator-Fiscal.

An exception to this rule is that fatal accidents in Scotland are statutorily made the subject of a public enquiry, conducted by the Sheriff with a jury of seven.

COT DEATH. (SUDDEN INFANT DEATH SYNDROME)

Frequency: One in 500
More common in boys than girls
More common in winter
Usually first 6 months of life, most within 1 year
Less common in breast fed babies

Action to take
As in sudden death. i.e. Establish death has occurred
Identify deceased
Examine body thoroughly, to exclude non-accidental death
    e.g. bruises, petechiae, burns, fractures
History from parents, symptoms, feeding habits, drugs given
Inform coroner
Coroner's officer deals with removal of body
Remove any drugs belonging to child

Leave address of:
Foundation for Study of Infant Deaths,
    5th Floor,
    Grosvenor Place,
    London SW1A 7HD
    Tel. 01-245-9421
    Evenings 01-748-7768

Follow up family
Listen and talk to parents and siblings
Involve Health Visitor in support of family
Advise mother on suppression of lactation if necessary
Discussion of grief and future pregnancies
Consider night sedation for parents if wanted or appropriate

SUDDEN DEATH

Procedure
Establish that death has occurred
Ascertain cause of death
Identify deceased
Discover circumstances from witnesses
Consider consulting colleagues or records
Consider informing police or coroner
Consider the removal of the body
Inform and discuss with relatives
Issue Death Certificate if possible

Police report
Limit report to information requested
Only record observed facts
Use drawings or photographs as appropriate
Make personal notes immediately
Do not interfere with police work

Brief statement of circumstances
Confirmation of death
Identity of deceased
Rigor mortis and body temperature
Cause of death
Position of body and state of clothing
Record of other relevant features
Retain any blood, tablets, vomitus

Check lists

KIDNEY DONOR

Ideal	**Acceptable**

Aged 5 to 50 years
Brain death from:
    Cerebral trauma
    Cerebral haemorrhage
    Proven primary brain
    tumour
    Cardiac arrest, cause
    known
	Aged 3 to 60 years
	All deaths without transmissible disease

Supported by a ventilator until the kidneys are removed as planned procedure	Most patients maintained on ventilators Death in circumstances which allow the kidneys to be removed and preserved within 45 minutes of cardiac arrest
Normal renal function and blood pressure No past history of either renal disease or hypertension	Moderate renal failure (blood urea less than 12 mmol/1) from either prerenal factors or tubular necrocis Oliguria for less than four hours Hypotension (systolic BP less than 80 mm Hg in an adult) for less than four hours Any kidney without transmissible disease which is capable of supporting life for five years
Exclude: AIDS or Hepatitis B antigenaemia before kidney is used	**Exclude:** AIDS or Hepatitis B antigenaemia before kidney is used
Sepsis	Generalized but not localized sepsis, e.g. bronchial aspirate
Malignancy other than primary brain tumour	Malignancy other than primary brain tumour

BLOOD DONOR

Absolute contraindications

Current infectious illness
Any medication (wait 3 days following aspirin ingestion)
Females under 8 stone in weight
Drug addiction
Disabled people in a wheelchair (due to insurance cover)
History of brucellosis, hepatitis B, syphylis or AIDS
Pregnancy (delay until the baby is a year old)
Recent travel to the tropics (wait 6 months)

Reasons for delaying donation

Glandular fever	2 years
Hepatitis A	1 year
Ear piercing	6 months
Tattooing	6 months
Acupuncture	6 months
Receiving a blood transfusion	6 months
Major surgery	6 months
Minor surgery	1 month approx.

Immunisations

Rubella	3 months
BCG, rabies, measles Oral polio, mumps Yellow fever	3 weeks
Hepatitis B vaccine	6 months
Anthrax, cholera Diphtheria, tetanus, flu Common cold, typhoid	1 week

Medicine and the law

CONSENT

Any treatment delivered without the consent of a patient is an assault, which may lead to an action for damages.

Consent may be either expressed (in writing or by word of mouth) or implied. The patient or a legally competent deputy should give *written* consent in the following circumstances:

Diagnostic procedures
Therapeutic procedures
Insurance examinations
Provision of medical reports
Research
Post mortem examinations
Bequest of tissues
Cases involving litigation or police

It is imperative that appropriate explanation is given to the patient regarding the proposed procedure and the onus rests with the practitioner to determine the capability of the patient to give valid consent.

In an emergency, where urgent treatment is required or the patient is unconscious, consent should be obtained from a near relative. Failing this the practitioner should render any treatment that he considers immediately necessary.

CONFIDENTIALITY

Confidentiality is implicit in the doctor-patient relationship. Breach of confidence is treated as professional misconduct by the General Medical Council.

Young patient
Patients below the age of 16 should normally have parental consent to all procedures. Certain circumstances may make this inadvisable or unsafe. Consider advice from colleagues or a defence society as appropriate.

Confidence of family and friends
It is the right of the patient, whether dead or alive, to keep his confidences with doctors secret from his family or friends if he so wishes.

Statutory duties
A doctor must report infectious and industrial diseases, and also births, stillbirths and deaths. He must return NHS records to the FPC on request but this does not include correspondence.

A doctor has a duty to give information to the police, on request, in relation to certain serious offences under the Road Traffic Act; the doctor should give only the patient's name and address, but no clinical details.

The prevention of Terrorism Act makes it an offence to fail to disclose information about terrorists.

Order of court
Refusal of a doctor to disclose confidential information on request may be in contempt of court. A doctor should first express reluctance to permit a breach of confidence. He should then request permission not to do so, or to do so only in writing.

Protection of the community
A patient, such as an epileptic driver, should first be encouraged to take appropriate action himself. If the doctor takes the initiative a defence society should first be consulted.

RECORDS AND RESPONSIBILITIES

Contractual duty

A GP has a contractual duty to keep proper records, for both legal and medical reasons. In the NHS, these should be on the forms provided by the Family Practitioner Committee. The records are owned by the Secretary of State.

Disclosure of records

Disclosure of records can be ordered by the courts not only when the doctor is directly involved, but a litigant can call for the production of his medical records if he is taking action against someone else and requires medical evidence to support his claim.

Disclosure of computerised information is governed by the Data Protection Act.

Vicarious liability

The evolution of the extended 'primary health care team' and computers has created new problems of professional confidence. The practitioner must decide to which team members and in what circumstances the medical records should be available. It must be stressed to all staff that any information they acquire about patients must be treated in absolute confidence.

PRESCRIBING

Registration with the GMC enables a practitioner to prescribe, possess and dispense drugs. The British National Formulary is published jointly by the BMA and the Pharmaceutical Society and gives full guidance on all aspects of prescribing. However, the following information may be of value.

The prescription
The prescriber has a legal responsibility for the drug prescribed even when acting on another's recommendation.

All prescriptions must be signed by hand.

All alterations must be initialled.

The 'NP' box (*Nomen Propium*) on the FP10 if deleted will indicate to the dispenser that no name is to be written on the label.

Any prescription should include:

    Patient's name and address – and age if under 12 years

    Name of the drug

    Dosage – use values above 1, e.g. 500 mg and not 0.5 g

    Frequency of dosage

    Total dose and volume – form and strength of preparation to be dispensed

    Signature and date

    Name and address of prescriber.

Prescription Form FP10

Non dispensing doctor	—white FP10, dispensed by chemist
Dispensing doctor	—white FP10, dispensed by doctor
	—blue FP10(D), dispensed by chemist
NHS Hospital out patients	—yellow FP10(HP)
HM Forces Dependants	—Buff FP10(S), dispensed by chemist

P R E S C R I B I N G–Continued

Labelling of containers
When dispensing drugs the label of the container should state:

The name of the preparation – if NP box is not deleted, or if NP box is not initialled in the case of a controlled drug. Alternatively, as a description according to the wording of the prescription.
The strength or concentration of the preparation.
The name of the patient.
The name of the Dispensing Partnership or Pharmacy.

Patient information
Name, dosage and timing of medicine
Storage and disposal of medicine
Expected cure or symptom relief
Degree of compliance necessary
Planned duration of treatment
Warning of potential side effects
Warning of potential interactions

PRESCRIBING CONTROLLED DRUGS

It is an offence to issue an incomplete prescription for a controlled drug and a pharmacist may not dispense such a prescription. The legal requirements under the Misuse of Drugs Regulations 1973 are that such prescriptions be:

Indelibly handwritten, signed and dated by the prescriber and include:

Name and address of patient
Dosage
Total quantity of drug in words and figures.

These requirements also apply to barbiturates

NHS PRESCRIBING
Certain drugs are not allowed to be prescribed on forms FP10 although they can still be prescribed privately.
A 'black list' is published by the DHSS and this lists all the products which are not available.

DRUGS FOR USE ABROAD
Drugs to be used abroad should be prescribed privately. Controlled drugs cannot be prescribed for patients leaving the country. It is an offence to carry controlled drugs abroad without a licence issued by the Secretary of State.

ACBS PRESCRIPTIONS
Some foods and toilet preparations may be prescribed under the NHS for conditions approved by The Advisory Committee on Borderline Substances. Such prescriptions should be endorsed ACBS.

MISUSE OF DRUGS REGULATIONS

The four schedules relate to the regulations governing the use of drugs.

The three classes relate to the harmfulness of the drugs and the degree of penalty if the drugs are misused.

Schedule 1
Exempts some common preparations containing codeine, dihydrocodeine, pholcodine, medicinal opium or morphine, cocaine and diphenoxylate from the stringent controls of Schedule 2.

Schedule 2
Imposes special requirements for prescribing cocaine, heroin, morphine (see above). Full dispensing record must be kept. Drugs must be kept in locked receptacle.

Schedule 3
Includes amphetamine derivatives. The requirements for Schedule 2 apply, but a register is not required.

Schedule 4
Special licence is required to prescribe this group of drugs which includes LSD, cannabis and other hallucinogens.

Class A
Includes morphine, opium, heroin, methadone, pethidine, cocaine, LSD, and injectable amphetamines.

Class B
Includes oral amphetamines, cannabis, codeine, pholcodine and phenmetrazine.

Class C
Includes methaqualaine and amphetamine derivatives.

PRESCRIBING FOR ADDICTS

A practitioner must have a special licence from the Home Secretary to prescribe the following drugs to addicts.

cocaine	dextromoramide
diamorphine	opium
morphine	methadone
dipipanone	oxycodone

Any of these drugs may be prescribed to addicts if there is an underlying organic disease.

NOTIFICATION OF ADDICTS

The Home Office keeps a register of those addicted to heroin, morphine, cocaine, pethidine, methadone, dextromoramide, dipipanone, and levorphanol.

The GP has access to this register by writing to the Chief Medical Officer or phoning 01-212-0335 or 01-212-6071.

A GP must notify the Chief Medical Officer of any person suspected to be addicted to the above drugs within 7 days. (Address: Drugs Branch, Romney House, Marsham Street, London SW1).

Notification must include:
Name and address of patient
Sex and date of birth
NHS number
Date of first attendance
Name(s) of the drug(s) of addiction.

Scotland and Northern Ireland
Notification to the Chief Medical Officer, Ministry of Health and Social Services, Dundonald House, Belfast.

In Scotland, drug addicts have to be notified to the Scottish Home and Health Department.

THERAPEUTIC ABORTION

The Abortion Act 1967 allows for two medical practitioners to certify the need for termination of pregnancy under the following circumstances:

1   That continuation of the pregnancy would involve risk to the life of the pregnant woman greater than if the pregnancy were terminated.
2   That it would involve risk of injury to the physical or mental health of the pregnant woman greater than if the pregnancy were terminated.
3   That it would involve risk of injury to the physical or mental health of any existing children of the pregnant woman's family greater than if the pregnancy were terminated.
4   That there is a substantial risk that if the child were born it would suffer from physical or mental abnormalities so as to be seriously handicapped.

There are exceptions to the above rules:
The operation and termination may be performed by a practitioner who forms the opinion in good faith that the termination is necessary, as an emergency, to save life or prevent grave permanent injury to the patient.

THERAPEUTIC ABORTION–Continued

Forms
Form HSA1 (green) signed by two medical practitioners to be kept in the patient's notes.

Form HSA2 signed by one medical practitioner for the emergency situation.

Form HSA3 (buff) is a notification of the operation and is sent to the DHSS and kept by them.

Place of termination
This must be an NHS hospital or an approved place.

Consent
This must be obtained from the patient. The husband's consent is not required legally.

With girls between sixteen and twenty-one years of age no consent is needed from the parents legally, but with the girl's permission, it is prudent to obtain their consent.

If the girl is under sixteen years of age and her wishes differ from those of her parents, then a defence society should be consulted.

Scotland and Northern Ireland
In Northern Ireland the Act does not apply.
In Scotland the forms are different for therapeutic abortion.

Medicine and the law

BEQUEST AND TRANSPLANTATION

Anatomy Act 1832
Those wishing to bequeath their bodies for dissection should be advised to contact the Professor of Anatomy at the nearest Medical School (in London, HM Inspector of Anatomy).

Human Tissues Act 1961
There are two ways organs can be obtained for transplant purposes:

1 'Contracting out'. After reasonable enquiry to exclude any objection by the deceased's relatives (or the deceased before death), the person in lawful possession of the body may authorise the use of any part of it for medical purposes.

2 'Contracting in'. When the deceased expressed the wish, the person in lawful possession of the body may accede to his request.

The consent of HM Coroner is required if an inquest is ordered, or is likely.

Corneal Grafting Act 1952
This Act permits the removal of eyes shortly after death in cases where the deceased had expressed willingness during life and the relatives are in agreement. Contact RNIB, 224 Great Portland Street, London W1.

WILLS

A doctor may be asked to examine a person who wishes to make a will to ascertain whether his mental state will permit a reasoned disposal of his property. He should only witness a patient's will if he is prepared to testify later to that patient's testamentary capacity. The patient should know what property he possesses and which people should reasonably benefit. He should know that he is making a will. As a witness the doctor will forego any legacy which might be received from the will.

SOLICITOR'S REPORT

Establish the purpose of the report and who is requesting it.
Write clearly and in layman's terms.
Information should relate only to questions asked.

    Hearsay evidence in a chronological account
    Patient's treatment and progress
    Objective findings
    Opinions on suffering and prognosis should be as objective
      as possible.

Retain a copy of the report for six years.
Statement of a proper fee.

Medicine and the law

WITNESS IN COURT

Establish what is expected in court
Establish what category of witness is required

Expert — with specialist knowledge
Professional — with particular knowledge of the case under discussion
Ordinary — with a citizen's responsibilities

Opinions previously given in written statements may be read out in court
Refer to notes made at the time with permission of the court
Remain as impartial as possible
Answer only what is asked and in simple language
Confine answers to fact rather than opinion
Admit to ignorance rather than elaborating the answers
Claim the appropriate statutory fee or negotiate the fee beforehand

The primary health care team

Aims
Health maintenance
Illness prevention
Assessment and management of illness
Rehabilitation
Supportive care

The 'nuclear team'
General practitioner
Treatment room sister
Dispenser
Receptionist
Practice manager
Health visitor
Community midwife
District nursing sister

The 'extended team'
Social worker
Care assistant
Home help
Family aid
Counsellor
Community psychiatric nurse
Geriatric health visitor
Chiropodist
Dietitian
Occupational therapist
Physiotherapist
Speech therapist
School nurse
School medical officer

TREATMENT ROOM SISTER or 'PRACTICE NURSE'

Employed by the practice or DHA. May require further training or supervision. The role may be extended to include:

Primary assessment	First contact, telephone advice
First aid and SRN	Accidents, dressings
procedures	Bandages, splints, plasters
	Infra-red treatment, syringing ears
	Assisting doctors, hospital liaison
	Allergy tests, audiograms
	Venepuncture, urinalysis, ECG
Minor operations	Suturing, warts, pessary changes
	Injections and abscesses
Clinics	'MOT'—health screening
	Diabetic, Hypertension
	Asthma, Cytology
	Obesity, Family planning
	Well-woman
Immunisations	Information, advice
	Assessment and injection
Health education	Information (patients and lay staff)
	Notice-board display
	Dietary and exercise advice
Counselling	
Stock-taking	Supplies dressings and drugs
and ordering	
Maintenance and	Surgical equipment
renewal	Resuscitation equipment,
	Laundry
	Disposal of sharps and clinical waste
Dispensing	

PRACTICE MANAGER

Employed by the practice or District Health Authority

Duties
Patients
Recognise patient's needs and wants
Patient Participation Group liaison
Complaints
Quality control

Primary health care team
Communication
Meetings and minutes
Welfare
Team development
Duty rotas

Liaison
Regional Health Authority, District Health Authority,
Family Practitioner Committee
Accountants and solicitors
Visitors

Training
New Practice Managers
Reception staff in-service training
New staff induction
Health education
Personal development

Administration
Health and Safety Officer
Book-keeping and accounts
Pensions, PAYE, SSP, NIC
Audit and statistics
Computer supervision
Quarterly reports
Stock-taking and equipment
Premises—furnishings and up-keep

RECEPTION STAFF

Employed by the practice or District Health Authority

Duties

Reception desk
First contact with patients and visitors
Administration of—appointments system
　　　　　　　　—treatment room
　　　　　　　　—clinics
Repeat prescriptions
Registrations

Telephone
Enquiries
Appointments
Advice

Filing
All patient contacts
Results and correspondence
Summaries and disease registers

Clerical
Computer registrations and recalls
Copy and audio-typing
Photocopying
Word processing

Health promotion
Appropriate use of health services
Notice-board information
Leaflet information

Housekeeping

HEALTH VISITOR

Employed by the District Health Authority and usually attached to a particular practice. Professionally independent.

They are SRN's with midwifery or obstetric experience and special training in health visiting.

Duties
Prevention of all types of ill health especially in young and old
Detection of ill health and surveillance of high risk groups
Recognition of need and mobilisation of resources
Health education
Provision of care including support in times of stress or illness
Duty is to visit all children, under 5, at least once

COMMUNITY MIDWIFE

Employed by District Health Authority usually 'group attached'. Professionally independent.

Duties
Antenatal clinic care
Antenatal classes
Intrapartum care
Postnatal care
Advice on infant feeding
Statutory duty to attend a mother for 10–28 days following delivery.

DISTRICT NURSING SISTER

Employed by District Health Authority and usually 'group attached'.

Practice in their own right and responsible for their own case-load. Sister leads a team which may include Staff nurses, SENs and Auxiliaries.

Nursing assessment of patients
Prescribe, direct and evaluate nursing care
Terminal care
Bereavement counselling
Rehabilitation towards patient independence
Health education
Liaison with other agencies
Facilitating financial and other benefits
Caring for the carers (supporting families)
Teaching
Personal development

DISPENSER

Employed by the practice

Duties
Dispensing
Recording prescriptions
Submission of prescriptions to PPA
Collecting prescription charges and payment to FPC
Stock control and ordering
Repeat prescriptions
Cleaning returned bottles
Dispensary security

STAFF CONTRACTS

Employment law is complex and legal advice should be sought when drawing up staff contracts. The BMA can advise. The major legislation is the Employment Protection (Consolidation) Act (1978).

The contract
Name and address of employer and employee
Date of start of employment
Job title and description
Place of work
Salary and method of payment. Incremental date and review
Hours of work. Overtime. Weekends and statutory holidays
Holiday entitlement and pay
Health and safety at work
Sickness or injury—terms and conditions, sick pay benefit
Maternity leave
Pension
Rights to notice and termination of employment
Details of any fixed contract
Disciplinary rules and procedures
Grievance procedure
Social security pensions—whether contracting out certificate
  is in force
Method of altering contract
Statement whether previous employment counts as part of
  continuous employment
Responsibility for personal property
Confidentiality of information
Professional Indemnity or Insurance

STATUTORY SICK PAY

Covers all employees sick for four or more days except those specified in the booklet *Employer's Guide to SSP* (N1 227) and notably those earning less than the lower weekly earnings limit for National Insurance.

Is payable for up to twenty-eight weeks thereafter sickness benefit becomes payable.

SSP is remibursed to the employer by witholding it from the monthly payments of National Insurance.

Employer must keep careful records of employee's days of absence.

Employee must complete form SC1 or employer's equivalent.

HIRING AND FIRING STAFF

Hiring
Establish a job description
Advertise—outline of job
　　　　　—qualifications required
　　　　　—Reply to include:
　　　　　　　age and sex
　　　　　　　curriculum vitae
　　　　　　　references
Short list applicants
Take up references
Arrange interviews
　　Intelligence
　　Experience
　　Special skills
　　Attainments
　　Interests
　　Circumstances, environment and family commitments
　　Attitudes to confidentiality
　　Ability to deal with people

Firing
Trade Union and Labour Relations Acts and Employment
　　Protection Acts outline procedures for industrial tribunals
　　and grounds for dismissal.
This excludes employees who:
　　work less than 8 hours a week
　　work less than 16 hours a week
　　　and employed for less than 5 years
　．have worked less than 26 weeks
Grounds for dismissal
Misconduct—employee should be given a stated number of
　　　　　　written warnings
　　　　　　—Act which leads to final dismissal must be
　　　　　　severe
　　　　　　—Gross misconduct would not require warning
Incapability—usually requires careful comparisons
Redundancy
Other substantial reasons

114

HEALTH AND SAFETY AT WORK

The most important pieces of legislation are:

Health and Safety at Work Act (1974)
Offices, Shops and Railway Premises Act (1963)
Employers Liability (Compulsory Insurance) Act (1969)

It is important to provide information, training and supervision to ensure health and safety at work

Issue written statement of general policy on health and safety to employees

Provide training in use of equipment

Provide standing orders and 'Policy File'

Ensure proper maintenance and safety of equipment

Keep Accident Book and Accident Report Forms, e.g. HMSO Book F2059 and Forms 2508

Ensure premises have Fire Certificate or meet approval of Fire Officer

Ensure staff Fire Training including evacuation

Display Fire Instructions

Ensure satisfactory toilet and washing facilities and supply of drinking water

Ensure satisfactory heating (16°C), lighting and ventilation. Display thermometer

There are legal requirements for floor space (40 ft^2/employee), breathing space (400 ft^3/employee) and seating when working

Provide storage for employees' personal effects

Ensure safe storage of drugs and chemicals (Medicines Act also applies)

Ensure safe disposal of waste, particularly clinical waste and 'sharps'

Display notices warning of any hazards

Consider appointing a 'Safety Officer'

Obtain Employer's Liability Insurance and display certificate

Seek advice of Crime Prevention Officer about security and Regional Medical Officer about security of drugs

Consider first-aid training for staff

Practice management

ALLOCATION TO A DOCTOR

A patient may apply to the FPC to be allocated to a doctor if he has been unable to register with practices in his area. The allocation committee will allocate to a specific doctor. There is usually an understanding that the specified doctor will keep the patient registered for a reasonable time.

CHANGING DOCTOR

Doctors
To remove a patient from his medical list the doctor applies in writing to the FPC who then inform the patient. Removal is effective 14 days after application is received.

Patients with medical cards
If a patient wishes to change doctors because of a change of address both the patient and the new doctor should sign Part A of the medical card, FP4. If the patient wishes to change doctors for any other reason, he may transfer at once if both the old and new doctors consent. In this case the new doctor and the patient sign Part A and the old doctor signs Part B. Alternatively the patient may write to the FPC stating that he intends to change doctors, enclosing his medical card. Transfer then takes 14 or more days.

Patients without medical cards
Form FP1 is filled in by the patient and doctor, stating that the card is missing, and sent to the FPC.

Dispensing
Form FP28A must also be completed for patients in a 'dispensing' area.

COMPLAINTS

Complaints against practitioners should normally be made to the FPC within 8 weeks. Complaints against hospitals should first to be taken to the hospital administratrom the DHA or the RHA, or via the Community Health Council. Complaints may then be taken to the Health Service Commissioner who is independent and whose job it is to investigate many complaints concerned with hospitals and other health services. Complaints should normally be made within 1 year. The HSC does not investigate any matter which the complainant could have brought before a tribunal or a court of law.

OVERSEAS VISITORS

Hospital services
People not ordinarily resident in the UK have to pay special statutory charges for most NHS hospital treatment unless specifically exempt. Generally 'ordinarily resident' means living lawfully in the UK voluntarily for a settled identifiable purpose and usually for more than six months.

Ambulance transport
There are no NHS charges for ambulance transport as provided to UK residents. Arrangements for repatriation should be made privately.

Family practitioner services
The hospital charges do not apply to FPS. The acceptance of a particular person, including an overseas visitor, remains at the discretion of a doctor within his conditions of service.

Overseas visitors requiring immediately necessary treatment owing to accident or emergency should be treated under the NHS (SFA para 4).

Most visitors from other EEC countries can be regarded as entitled to NHS treatment except when they have come specifically for treatment—in which case they should generally have the prior approval of their insurance institution and should be able to produce Form E112.

FPS charges (including prescription charges)
Overseas visitors are liable to the statutory charges for FPS services on the same basis as UK residents.

Domiciliary nursing
Is provided to overseas visitors on the same basis as to UK residents without additional charges.

OVERSEAS VISITORS - continued.

Reciprocal arrangements
The UK has reciprocal arrangements with the following countries for treatment of their nationals when the need for treatment arises during a visit to the UK.

Anguilla	Isle of Man
Australia	Malta
Austria	Montserrat
British Virgin Isles	New Zealand
Bulgaria	Norway
Channel Islands	Poland
Czechoslovakia	Portugal
Falkland Islands	Romania
Finland	St Helena
German Democratic Republic	Sweden
Gibraltar	Turks & Caicos Is.
Hong Kong	USSR
Hungary	Yugoslavia
Iceland	

Patients from other countries or those who have come to the UK specifically to obtain treatment without entitlement may be treated privately.

Private treatment
GPs should clearly advise patients of their entitlements under reciprocal arrangements and whether they are being treated privately or under the NHS. Patients referred to hospital should be advised to enquire at the hospital about their detailed entitlement and liabilities.

Further information
Consult FPN 353 or contact hospital or FPC administrator.

Practice management

DISPENSING PRACTICES

General practitioners may provide a dispensing service for their patients when authorised to do so. The following conditions apply:

The area must be designated as 'rural' by the FPC

The patient must live more than a mile from a chemist

Outline consent must be obtained from the Rural Dispensing Committee set up under the 'Clothier' report. This is a central committee and applications are made through the FPC

The patient must complete FP28A

Method of payment
The Capitation Fee System has been abolished

Drug tariff method
The basic price or 'net ingredient cost'
An on-cost allowance of the net cost
A container allowance per prescription
A dispensing fee
Appropriate FP10's must be used—see page 131

ORGANISING A DISPENSARY

Design and layout
Security and controlled drugs
Staff training and supervision
Tablet counters, bottles, labels
Ordering and stock control
Documentation
Claiming fees
Financial audit
Prescription charges
Collection and transport
Repeat prescriptions
Drug record in case notes
Drug audit and formulary
Relationship with pharmacists
Relationship with suppliers
Drug information service
Patient information cards

TREATMENT ROOM

Examination
Sphygmomanometer
Stethoscope and foetal
   stethoscope
Ophthalmoscope,
   auroscope, torch,
Scales
Height measure
Tape measure
Bunsen burner or spirit
   lamp

PR tray and proctoscope,
   sigmoidoscope
PV tray and specula
Patella hammer
Tuning fork
Laryngeal mirror
Nasal speculum
Vision charts
Colour vision charts
Audiometer
Fetal ultrasound

Investigation
ECG
Peak flow meter
Microscope and slides
Urine cell counting
   chamber
Haemoglobinometer
Blood Sugar Meter
Dipsticks

Centrifuge
Refrigerator with
   freezer compartment
ESR equipment
Needles and syringes
Swabs
Magnifying goggles

Treatment
Suturing equipment
Dressings and bandages
Wax hook
Ear syringe
Lotion thermometer
Dressing tongs
Gloves
CO_2 snow apparatus
Various forceps
Spongeholder
Clip removers
Suture scissors
Ring cutter

Bandage scissors
Scalpel
Razor
Orange sticks
Airway
Anaesthetic equipment
Resuscitation equipment
Eye tray
Diathermy
Autoclave and steriliser
IUCD equipment

CONSULTING ROOM

Size

Combined consulting/examination room —minimum 11 m^2
or consulting room —minimum 9.5 m^2
with examination room —minimum 4.5 m^2

Construction

Sound proof
Hand-washing facilities with running water
Privacy for patients
Desk and chairs
Couch and step
Modesty blanket
Heating and lighting
Shelves and storage
Telephone
Patient call system

Equipment

Diagnostic and administrative (see p. 158)
Reference books
Rectal tray and proctoscope
Vaginal tray and speculae
Peak flow meter and placebo inhalers
Eye charts
Colour vision charts
Paediatric assessment equipment
Height rule
Weighing scales
Toy box
Box for notes
In/out tray
Dictation equipment
Rubber stamps and pad
Waste-paper basket and sharps box
Note pads and stationary supplies
Full range of forms

LOCUMS

Employing a locum

Overall responsibility for patient care remains that of the employing doctor.

Ensure that the locum is registered with the GMC and a medical defence organisation.

Establish his requirements for accommodation and transport.

Written agreement covering:

Duration of locum and length of notice

Payment, car and other allowances

Board and lodging, single or family accommodation

Workload, extent of duties, nights and weekends

The BMA can advise on current rates of pay.

CONTRACTING OUT – out of hours duties

Applicaton

To the FPC. 3 months notice is required (3 months is also required for termination of contracting out). The application may be accompanied by a recommendation for a particular doctor.

Selection

By the LMC and the FPC of the doctor recommended or a doctor from the supplementary list of the FPC.

Responsibility

It is the responsibility of the contracted doctor only to carry out duties that were requested out of hours and to ensure effective continuity of care.

It is the responsibility of the general practitioner to inform his patients of the change in 'on call' services.

Remuneration

A doctor employed from the supplementary list of the FPC is entitled to the supplementary capitation fees, the supplementary practice allowance and the night visit fees.

ASSESSING A DEPUTISING SERVICE

Services offered
Details of contracts
Costing of services

Medical personnel
Selection procedure used
Standard of practice required
Suitable for obstetric and GP hospital duties
Adequate numbers for the population served

Supporting Staff
Experience of telephonists and drivers

Priority of calls
Effective assessment of urgency

Response to calls
A doctor should be involved in the giving of any advice

Communications
Adequate radio or telephone links with control room, the
doctor, and the patient's own GP as necessary

Continuity of care
Effective reporting of all cases and the action taken to GP

Records
Full records of all telephone calls made to the deputising
service

AGE–SEX REGISTER

Administration
Population profile
FPC claims
Previous registrations and 'turnover'

Screening 'call and recall'
Cytology
Blood pressure

Immunisation programmes
Rubella
Tetanus
Polio

Disease register
Chronic diseases, e.g. hypertension, diabetes
Disabled patients
'At risk' patients
Rare clinical conditions
Overdose and self-injury patients

Geriatric serveillance

Bereavement file
Bereavement visits
Cancer register

COMPUTERS IN PRIMARY CARE

Administration
Patient register
Word processor
Dispensary stock-control
Staff salaries
Finance

Age–sex register

Disease register
'At risk' disease groups
Morbidity register

Prescriptions
Repeat prescription print-outs
Drug interactions

Patient recall
Preventive care
Item of service payments
Cervical cytology screening
BP screening

Patient data base
New patient questionnaires
Past medical history
Relevant family history

Research
Case finding
Controls
Self-audit

Education
Reference 'book' for medical information
Information source for teaching

RCGP COLOUR CODES

Colour	Group	Overprinted	Notes
Red	Hypersensitivity	HYPERS. TO	Drug sensitivities, severe toxic reactions, idiosyncrasies, major allergies
Brown	Diabetes	DIAB.	Types I and II
Yellow	Epilepsy	EPIL.	
Green	Tuberculosis	TB.	Active, arrested or cured
Blue	Hypertension	HYPERTEN.	By agreed criteria for the therapy or surveillance
White	Long term maintenance therapy	LTM THERAPY	E.g. steroids, thyroid, Vit B_{12}, antibiotics
Black	Attempted suicide		
Chequered	Measles	MEAS.	
Pink			
Pale yellow			
Light blue			For individual doctor's use

IN THE NOTES

Summary Card

Name	Sex
Address	Date of birth
Telephone number	Marital status
Occupation	Partner's occupation
Allergies	Height
Immunisation status	Ideal weight
Smoking	Parity
Alcohol	Contraception record
Cytology record	Chronic illness (colour codes)
Family history	Colour coding

Serial recordings of weight and blood pressure

Medical History—
in chronological order
Recurrent diseases
Persistent diseases
Severe diseases
Accidents
Fractures
Hospital admissions
Operations

Life events—
in chronological order
Births
Marriage and divorce
Deaths
Leaving home
New jobs and unemployment
Moving home
Successes and disappointments

Continuation card abbreviations

A	Attendance of patient
V	Visit to patient
C	Certificate
NV	Night visit
ET	Emergency treatment
T or P	Advice by 'phone

Practice management

CERTIFICATES

MED 3
: Standard statement of illness by the doctor
To be issued after 7 days of illness
Vague diagnosis—submit supplementary MED 6
Not to be issued retrospectively
Not to be issued without examination

MED 5
: Special statement by the doctor
Use when MED 3 is inappropriate
For a previous illness if patient was seen but no certificate was issued
For an illness verified by another doctor

MED 6
: Special statement to RMO
Explanation of a 'vague diagnosis' on MED 3
Explanation of the true diagnosis, if not known by the patient

RM7
: Referral to the RMO
For second opinion as to whether patient is fit for work

SC1
: Self certification by the patient to be completed after four days' illness
Required for the first seven days' of illness
Also used as the claim for for SSP, sickness benefit and invalidity benefit

CW8
: Certificate of pregnancy

MAT B₁
: Certificate of expected confinement issued after 26 weeks
Submitted with BM4 to the DHSS by the patient

MAT B₂
: Certificate of confinement

Northern Ireland
In Northern Ireland names of certificates differ slightly

NHS FORMS

NHS forms can be obtained from the Family Practitioner Committee by completing Form FP30A.

Completed NHS forms should be sent to the local FPC or to the FPC appropriate to a patient's area if not on a practitioner's own list.

General medical

FP4   Medical Card.

FP5/6   Medical Record Envelope (male and female).

FP7/8   Continuation Card   (male and female).

FP22 A-E   Request for FPC to return patient's notes. Application used when a patient has left an area, emigrated or died.

FP28A   Supply of Medicines and Appliances Prescribed by the Doctor ('Dispensing Form').

FP58   Application for inclusion on doctor's list (babies only).

FP69   Notice of removal of patient from doctor's list. To be effective within 6 months.

FP92   Prescription charge exemption certificate.

MCW01   Co-operation record card for maternity patients.

MCWO2A   Envelope for record card for maternity patients.

Treatment

FP10   Prescription Form.

FP19   Record of treatment of temporary resident. For patients staying in the area between 24 hours and 3 months.

FP31   General anaesthetics service claim form.

FP32   Emergency treatment claim form. For patients staying in the area for less than 24 hours.

FP82   Application for arrest of dental haemorrhage.

FP106   Immediately necessary treatment.

N H S F O R M S—Continued

Services

FP24 — Maternity Medical Services. Certificate and claim for payment applicable for doctors on the obstetric list. This form is also used for emergency maternity services including treatment of miscarriage.

FP24A — Maternity Medical Services. Certificate and claim for payment applicable for doctors not on the obstetric list.

FP73 — Vaccination and immunisation claim.

FP74 — Cervical cytology certificate and claim. For patients aged over 35 years having cytology at 5 yearly intervals.

FP1001 — Application for contraceptive services. Annual application.

FP1002 — Contraceptive services – fitting of intra-uterine device.

FP1003 — Contraceptive services – treatment of person temporarily absent from home.

Allowances

FP16	Application for inclusion on the Medical List. This constitutes the legal contract with the FPC. It also includes application for maternity and contraceptive services.
FP16A	Application for filling a practice vacancy in reply to an advertised vacancy.
FP30A	Requisition by doctor for certificates, prescriptions and other claim forms from the FPC.
FP36	Claim for rota/late duty service.
FP45	Trainee Practitioner Scheme. Claim for payment to pay the trainee's allowance.
FP70A	Postgraduate training allowance claim.
FP75	Application for leave payment.
FP76	Application for designated area allowance.
FP77	Application for group practice allowance.
FP78	Application for vocational training addition.
FP79	Application for seniority allowance.
FP80	Application for assistants allowance.
FP81	Application for night visit fee.
FC21	Remuneration of assistant practitioner.
ANC 1-6	Ancillary staff records and reimbursement.
RAN1–3	Related ancillary staff.
PREM2	Annual claim for payment of rent and rates.
LOC1	Application for additional payments during practitioner's sickness.

Scotland and Northern Ireland

Certain of the forms listed above have different numbers in Scotland and Northern Ireland. For precise details, contact Health Boards as forms change frequently.

CERTIFICATION

Abortion before 28th week
No notification required. No certificate required.

Stillbirth
Certificate to be signed by doctor and midwife. Also Registrar must be notified by parent, guardian, or house owner within 42 days (21 days in Scotland).

Neonatal death
Certificate to be signed by registered doctor if death occurs within the first 28 days of life.

Live births
No certification but notification to the DHA by hospital, midwife or doctor within 36 hours. Also notification to Registrar by parent guardian, or house owner within 42 days.

Death
Certificate may be signed by the doctor if the deceased has been seen by him within 14 days and there is no doubt of the diagnosis.

If the deceased has not been seen within 14 days or only after the death has occurred, the Registrar must inform the Coroner.

If the diagnosis is in doubt, report the death to the Coroner who may then authorise certification. In this case the appropriate box on the reverse of the certificate should be completed.

Scotland and Northern Ireland
In Scotland and Northern Ireland the regulations may differ.

CREMATION FORMS

A   Request for cremation completed by close relative of the deceased.

B   First medical certificate completed by attendant doctor.

C   Confirmatory medical certificate completed by an independent doctor registered more than 5 years, having consulted the attendant doctor and examined the body.

D   Replaces forms B and C when it is completed by a pathologist following a post-mortem examination.

E   Replaces forms B and C when it is completed by the Coroner.

F   Authority to cremate. It is completed by the Medical Referee for Cremation.

NHS PAYMENTS

The System of Payments for general practitioners under the National Health Service is detailed in the statement of Fees & Allowances (The Red Book).

Basic practice allowance & additions for:

Designated areas
Group practice
Seniority

Vocational training
Employing an assistant

Standard capitation fees depending on patients age

Payments of Out-of-hours responsibilities

Supplementary practice allowance
Supplementary capitation fees
Night visit fees

Fees for items of service for:

Vaccinations and immunisations
Contraceptive services
Cervical cytology
Maternity services
Temporary residents
Emergency treatment
Services as anaesthetist
Arrest of dental haemorrhage
Immediately necessary treatment

Postgraduate training
Trainee scheme
Doctors' retainer scheme
Initial practice allowance
Rural practice
Supply of drugs and
   appliances

Practising in inducement areas

Special arrangements for:

Sickness
Confinement
Prolonged study leave

Arrangements for reimbursement for:

Rent and rates
Ancillary staff
Related ancillary staff

Improvement grants
Group practice loans

FEES FOR SERVICES

The British Medical Association publishes details of the statutory, agreed and recommended fees for a wide variety of part-time medical services.

Services for which fees may be charged
Reports for attendance allowance
Insurance examinations and reports
Cremation certificates
Examination of drivers and pilots
Pre-employment medicals
Incapacity certificates (other than National Insurance)
Services to the Police, Coroner or Courts
Immunisation for travel abroad where a fee is not payable by the Family Practitioner Committee

Services for which fees may not be charged
Death and stillbirth certificates
Maternity certificates
National Insurance certificates

RENT AND RATES

The rent and rates of practice accommodation is reimbursible
  by the FPC if certain criteria are met. Full details are set out
  in the SFA (Red Book)
Rates, levied by local authorities or water authorities will be
  reimbursed.
Rent can be calculated in a number of ways.
  Paid to a landlord or local authority
  Notional rent for owner—occupiers
  Cost rent for new separate purpose built premises or their
    equivalent. This is a rent related to the cost of building
    work rather than the current market rent.

Improvement grants
Are available towards the cost to doctors of improving existing
medical practice premises and can be one-third of the cost of
approved work and professional statutory fees.

Source of income
There are now many sources of loans for GP's—banks, some
building societies and the GPFC—which offer loans and
lease-back scheme.
  Any GP considering new premises or improvements is
advised to consult his FPC and specialist RMO (DHSS).

INCOME TAX

Your accountant may require the following information to prepare your annual tax return:

Income tax return form
Form P60
Form P45
Book of accounts
Details of pensions
Pay slips
Unearned income—tax dividends
        —building societies
        —deposit accounts and income not taxed at
          source
        —royalties, copyright fees
Personal expenses—secretarial expenses
        —stationery and postage
        —renewals and repair of equipment
        —laundry and cleaning
        —proportion of household expenses
        —on-call telephone answering
General expenses
Travelling expenses
Motoring expenses
Life assurance and pension annuity policies
Mortgage statement
Rent received and expenses incurred
Payments under deed of covenant
Charges against income
Professional subscriptions
Medical books and equipment bought
Alimony/maintenance
Marital status
Children born during year
Dependant relatives

ACCOUNTING SYSTEMS

Discuss with your accountant a system suitable for your practice

Main account book for bank transactions
Cash book—income
Cash book—payments
Wages book
Fees ledger
Purchase invoice file
Income statements file
Receipts file
Bank and building society statements
Cheque stubs
Paying-in books

Columns in main account book

Expenditure
Date
Narrative/description
Cheque No.
Salaries—staff eligible FP reimbursement
Salaries—other staff
Partners' drawings
Light and heat
Phones and communications
Rent and rates

Insurance
Drugs and medical supplies
Stationary and printing
Locum fees
Petty cash
Cleaning and laundry
Repairs and renewals
Capital
Sundries

Income
Date
Narrative
Ref. No.
FPC
Dispensing
Medical insurance and reports
Private patients
Outside appointments

Vocational training

ROYAL COLLEGE OF GENERAL PRACTITIONERS
(14 Princes Gate, London SW7 IPU)

Aims
To encourage, foster and maintain the highest standards in general practice.

Membership
Full membership by pass in MRCGP examination

Associate membership available to those who have not taken or are ineligible to take the examination.

The MRCGP examination is held twice a year and consists of written papers and oral examinations.

Eligibility
Fully registered for at least four years, of which two have been in general practice or completion of a vocation training course or approved equivalent

Benefits
Membership constitutes the only postgraduate qualification in primary care in the UK

Quality initiative— Fostering good general practice

Accommodation and facilities for functions

Faculties organise a range of functions, meetings and conferences throughout the country

Electronic technology department—computers

Press Office—deals with the media

International affairs

Working parties have been set up involving many topics

College library—a major reference library

Information service—information on physical and organisational aspects of practice. Publishes record cards for sale

Online search—computerised services to researchers

Prestel

Publications—journal, occasional papers, booklets, and RCGP Members Reference Book

Education—courses, examinations and educational research

Research—research units and projects

HIPPOCRATIC OATH

'I swear by Apollo the Physician, by Aesculapius, by Hygieia, by Panacea, and by all the gods and goddesses, making them my witnesses, that I will carry out according to my ability and judgement, this oath and this indenture. To hold my teacher in this art equal to my own parents; to make him partner in my livelihood; when he is in need of money to share mine with him; to consider his family as my own brothers, and to teach them this art, if they want to learn it, without fee or indenture; to impart precept, oral instruction, and all other instruction to my own sons, the sons of my teacher, and to pupils who have taken the physicians' oath, but to nobody else. I will use treatment to help the sick according to my ability and judgement, but never with a view to injury and wrongdoing. Neither will I administer a poison to anybody when asked to do so, nor will I suggest such a course. Similarly I will not give to a woman a pessary to cause abortion. But I will keep pure and holy both my life and my art. I will not use the knife, not even, verily, on sufferers from stone, but I will give place to such as are craftsmen therein. Into whatsoever houses I enter, I will enter to help the sick, and I will abstain from all intentional wrongdoing and harm, especially from abusing the bodies of man or woman, bound or free. And whatsoever I shall see or hear in the course of my profession, as well as outside my profession in my intercourse with men, if it be what should not be published abroad, I will never divulge, holding such things to be holy secrets. Now if I carry out this oath, and break it not, may I gain forever reputation among all men for my life and for my art; but if I transgress it and forswear myself, may the opposite befall me.'

DECLARATION OF GENEVA

At the time of being admitted as a Member of the Medical Profession:

I solemnly pledge myself to consecrate my life to the service of humanity;

I will give to my teachers the respect and gratitude which are their due;

I will practise my profession with conscience and dignity;

The health of my patient will be my first consideration;

I will respect the secrets which are confided in me;

I will maintain by all the means in my power the honour and the noble traditions of the medical profession;

My colleagues will be my brothers;

I will not permit considerations of religion, nationality, race, party politics or social standing to intervene between my duty and my patient;

I will maintain the utmost respect of human life from the time of conception; even under threat, I will not use my medical knowledge contrary to the laws of humanity.

I make these promises solemnly, freely and upon my honour.

PRIORITY OBJECTIVES

Patient care

Problem definition
Recognise common physical, psychological and social
 problems
Assess patients beliefs, effects on daily living, effect on
 psychological state, patient's expectations of the doctor
Understand the principles of problem definition
Cope with own anxieties

Management
Chose with the patient appropriate management
Involve other members of the team
Use records effectively
Prescribe appropriately
Manage life events and crises
Provide appropriate care and support
Make appropriate referrals
Involve and educate the patient
Be aware of the cost

Emergency care
Diagnose and initially manage all acute emergencies

Prevention
Understand the principles of case finding, health education
 and screening
Understand systems for information handling
Provide effective preventive services

Communication

Patients
Consultants tasks (see p. 56)

Partners, team and other professionals
Understand the roles of other professionals
Understand meetings
Understand others' needs
Use personal resources appropriately

PRIORITY OBJECTIVES – Continued

Organisation

The practice
Manage the practice effectively
Monitor practice activity
Solve problems appropriately
Understand the NHS contract and regulations
Understand legal and financial aspects of practice
Use appropriate technology
Manage change and innovation

Personal organisation
Manage time
Delegate appropriately

Community
Respond to the community's health needs
Participate in community affairs

Professional values
Be aware of personal values
Recognise social, cultural and organisational factors that
    affect work
Maintain ethical principles
Respond to others with tolerance, respect and flexibility
Submit to critical peer-review
Maintain physical and mental health
Balance personal and professional commitments
Accept appropriate responsibility

Personal and professional growth

Identify personal strengths and weakness
Recognise changing needs in others
Define own educational needs
Adapt to change
Be aware of personal limiting factors

Printed by permission of the Oxford Region Course Organisers and Regional
    Advisers Group from occasional paper No. 30 (RCGP), 'Priority Objectives
    for General Practice Vocational Training'.

VOCATIONAL TRAINING ADDITION*

The Addition is payable to Principals who satisfy the FPC that they have undertaken the appropriate training. This is payable until the first seniority payment is due.

Vocational training requirements

A period of training of four or more years is required from the date of provisional registration. This comprises the equivalent of twelve months in a NHS general practice as a trainee and a minimum of three years in hospital posts in NHS hospitals or with HM forces. At least one year of the hospital posts must include two or more of the following specialties:

General medicine
Chest medicine
Traumatic surgery or accident and/or emergency work
Obstetrics and gynaecology
Paediatrics
Psychiatry
Geriatrics
Otorhinolaryngology
Dermatology
Ophthalmology
Anaesthesia

An alternative is a special course arranged by or with a university including experience in hospitals and general practice.

The doctor must hold a certificate of prescribed or equivalent experience.

Full information may be found in the NHS Statement of Fees and Allowances.

* Information from 'The Statement of Fees and Allowances payable to General Medical Practitioners' by permission of the Department of Health and Social Security.

SELECTING A VOCATIONAL TRAINING SCHEME

Seek the advice of the Regional Adviser, the local course organiser and past and present trainees on the scheme.

Organisation
Sequence and duration of job rotation
Flexibility in jobs offered
Compatability with previous experience
Attitudes to women and part-timers
Attitudes to change after starting course or early cessation
Contact with GP trainers whilst in hospital jobs
Feedback and trainee participation in organisation
Opportunity to visit prior to selection
The Contract

Hospital jobs
Experience and training offered and relevance to GP
Duties, rotas, on-call arrangements
Opportunities for further diplomas and degrees
Time off for GP or other teaching
Accommodation offered

GP
Characteristics of training practices (see p. 152)
Facilities offered to trainee
Characteristics of trainers and their partners
Location of practices and travelling involved
Travel and telephone arrangements

Teaching
Organisation of time and subjects
Training methods and attitudes
Attitudes to additional study leave or courses
Library and reference facilities

CURRICULUM VITAE

Name	Qualifications
Address	Age
Telephone No.	Marital status
School	Scholarships and prizes
University	Degrees, distinctions and prizes
Postgraduate experience	Hospital jobs
	Diplomas and degrees
	Publications and research
	Other appointments
	General practice experience

Medical interests
Career interests
Medical societies and communities
Other interests

GMC registration number
Defence Society membership
Certificate of prescribed or equivalent experience
Name and address of referees

Accompanying letter
Nationality
Religion
Health
Family details
Availability

THE TRAINEE CONTRACT

The trainee should agree on terms of service with the trainer. This may take the form of a contract or letter of employment which should include at least the following:

Dates of commencement and duration of contract
Notice required for termination of contract
An undertaking by the trainer to teach and advise
Salary and frequency of payment as in 'Statement of Fees and Allowances'
Leave: holiday, illness, maternity and study leave
Medical equipment to be provided by trainer
Provision of car or car allowance
Membership of a Defence Organisation
Full registration with GMC
Working hours, night and weekend duties
Accommodation—if applicable
Settlement of disputes by arbitration

The terms of the contract should be subject to Terms of Service for Doctors (as set out in NHS General Medical Services) and the Employment Protection Acts).
The BMA and Defence Societies have produced model contracts for trainees and assistants joining practices.

PAYMENT OF TRAINEES

The trainee undertaking hospital jobs is paid by the Health Authority as any other junior hospital doctor under NHS General Whitley Council conditions of service. When undertaking the trainee year in general practice, the trainee is employed by his trainer. He is not self employed. The trainer must not pay the trainee any salary or emolument in excess of the amounts specified in the SFA.

The trainee pays the relevant employee's portion of the National Insurance and Superannuation. This is usually deducted at source.

The Employment Protection & Safety at Work legislation applies to trainees.

The SFA should be consulted as it details:

Rates of trainee salary, weightings and increments

Allowances for motoring expenses

Reimbursement of telephone installation charges

Reimbursement of removal, house purchase, storage and other expenses

Reimbursement of travelling expenses and subsistence involved in obtaining accommodation

Reimbursement of losses arising from educational arrangements for children

Allowances during searches for accommodation

Reimbursement of miscellaneous expenses on moving

Allowances for continuing commitments relating to previous accommodation

Payment of rent of unoccupied property

Payment of expenses when on call

Payment of excess rent

Payment of interview expenses for traineeships

Payments during sickness. During sickness lasting less than two weeks the trainee is usually paid by the trainer less SSP deductions and this should not affect recognition of training. For longer than this, consult FPC

Maternity leave

Examinations: travelling expenses and subsistence is reimbursable but *not* the examination fees

EXPENSES AND SUBSISTENCE
(Section 63)

Under Section 63 of the Health Services and Public Health Act (1968), expenses and a subsistence allowance are claimable for principals, assistants, trainees and ancillary staff attending postgraduate meetings and courses approved by the University Postgraduate Deans.

Trainees must obtain approval from their postgraduate dean before attending courses outside their own region.

The rate of reimbursement increases periodically. Claim forms are issued whilst attending the course and signature of the attendance register is mandatory.

The limit on claims per year varies from region to region.

Forms

GPRC 3 for principals
GPRC 5 for assistants
GPRC 8 for trainees
GPRC 13 for trainees for postgraduate examination expenses

Scotland and Northern Ireland
In Scotland and Northern Ireland the forms are different.

SELECTING A PRACTICE

The practice organisation
List size and characteristics
Appointments system
On-call work
Workload
Work share
Annual, sick, maternity and study leave
Telephone cover
Age, sex and disease registers
Record systems
Research
Teaching
Outside interests
The primary health care team

The practice facilities
Premises: health centre, surgeries, ownership
Treatment room
Dispensary
Equipment
Computer
Library
Teaching aids

The partners
Ages and sexes, of partners
Medical interests and qualifications
Ethical and moral issues
Decision making
Partners' motivation
Attitudes to innovation
Attitudes to the incoming partner
Priorities claimed for seniority
Outside interests
Spouses and families
Politics and religion

SELECTING A PRACTICE—Continued

Finance
Time to parity
Method of payment to parity
Distribution of income
NHS and private income
Inspect accounts
Tax liability
Cost of joining practice
Future expenses

The practice area
Local hospitals
Consultants
Waiting lists
Liaison with other practices
Laboratories and paramedical services
Postgraduate education
Local medical politics

The community
Housing
Transport
Shops
Schools
Cultural and leisure facilities
Proposed building and development
Local politics

FORMS ON ENTRY TO PRACTICE

The forms required on entry to practice will vary between FPCs. Always consult the FPC Administrator at the earliest opportunity.

Applicants for single-handed vacancies must apply on the forms specified by the FPC—FP16A.

Applicants for vacancies in partnerships should apply as advertised.

All successful candidates should check that FPC and Medical Practices Committee approval is complete before entering any commitments—particularly financial.

FORMS TO BE COMPLETED
(where appropriate)

Application for inclusion on medical list	(FP16)
Application for addition to basic practice allowance for vocational training	(FP78)
Application for NHS superannuation scheme	(SS14(RD))
Declaration of partnership	(FPC pro forma)
Declaration of time spent in GP (for BPA)	(FPC pro forma)
Authorisation of voluntary levy for local medical committee	(FPC pro forma)
Authorisation for rural dispensing compensation fund	(FPC pro forma)
Authorisation to banks for crediting NHS remuneration by FPC	(FPC pro forma)
Application for inclusion in obstetric list	(FPC pro forma)
Application for group practice allowance	(FP77)
Application for designated area allowance	(FP76)
Application for seniority allowance	(FP79)
Application for initial practice allowance	(FPC pro forma)
Application for postgraduate training allowance	(FP70A)

DOCUMENTATION ON ENTRY TO PRACTICE (as appropriate)

GMC—certificate of full registration (current)

Defence Society—certificate of membership (current)

Birth certificate

Certificate of prescribed or equivalent experience issued by JCPTGP (14 Princes Gate, London SW7) or statement of grounds of exemption (with supporting evidence)

National Insurance number

P45 or statement of tax position

Certificate of training in family planning (JCC)

Evidence of postgraduate obstetric qualification or experience or previous inclusion in an FPC Obstetric List as detailed in application form for inclusion in obstetric list

Evidence of receipt of seniority payments/date first inclusion in a medical list

THE PARTNERSHIP CONTRACT

Partnership contracts are complex and a solicitor's advice should be sought. It should cover the following topics as appropriate:

Who is to form the partnership
Commencement date and duration of contract
Arrangements and grounds for termination of contract
Details of practice premises and equipment
Terms of rental or purchase
Division of income and arrangements to parity
Financial responsibility for personal and partnership expenses, debts and tax, shares of assets and gifts
Definition of income to go to practice or partner (including vocational training and seniority payments).
Superannuation arrangements
Restrictions on private residency and distance from practice
Restrictions on other business or medical commitments
Membership of Defence Society and medical registration
Procedure in case of removal from medical register
Terms of employment of staff
Arrangements concerning communications and telephones
Retirement of partner
Selection of a new partner
Length and priority of holidays, study leave
Arrangements about representative or outside appointments
Engagement of locums
Arrangements in case of Military Service
Allowable absences and maternity leave
Arrangements on death or chronic illness of partners
Personal debts not to be secured against partnership assets
Settlement of disputes by arbitration

NOTES

Consulting room bookshelf

Abortion Law, Medical Protection Society

ABPI Data Sheet Compendium, Datapharm Publications Ltd, 12 Whitehall London SW1A 2DU

British National Formulary (BNF), British Medical Association and the Pharmaceutical Society of Great Britain

The Business of General Practice (prepared by General Practitioner and Medeconomics for the General Medical Services Committee)

The Casualty Officer's Handbook (Ellis, M.), Butterworth

Childrens' Developmental Progress (Sheridan, M.D.), National Federation for Educational Research

A Colour Atlas of Dermatology (Levene, G.M. & Calman, C.D.), Wolfe Medical

Drug Tarrif (DHSS), HMSO

First Aid Manual, St John Ambulance Association/St Andrew's Ambulance Association/British Red Cross Society

The General Practitioner's Year Book (Lansdell, D.A.E., ed.), Winthrop

A Guide to Social Services, Family Welfare Association

Handbook of Contraceptive Practice (DHSS), HMSO

Handbook of Medical Ethics, British Medical Association

Health on Holiday (Dick, G.), British Medical Association

Immunisation against Infectious Disease (DHSS), HMSO

Legal Aspects of Medical Practice (Knight, B.), Churchill Livingstone

List of Fees, British Medical Association

Medical Aspects of Fitness to Drive, Medical Commission on Accident Prevention

Medical Emergencies & Treatment (Robinson, R.O.), Wm. Heinemann

Medical Evidence for Social Security and Statutory Sick Pay Purposes (DHSS), HMSO

MIMS, Medical Publications Ltd

MIMS Colour Index, Medical Publications Ltd

Notes on Clinical Side Room Methods (Medical Education Committee). Churchill Livingstone

Ocular Emergencies (Richards, A.B.), Smith & Nephew Pharmaceuticals Ltd

OTC Index, Medical Publications Ltd

Paediatric Vade Mecum (Wood, B.S.B.), Lloyd-Luke

Patient's Rights (National Consumer Council), HMSO

A Practical Guide to Mental Health Law (Gostin, L.), MIND

Pulse Blue Book: Forms and Fees (Bowles, D.), Morgan-Grampian

Statement of Fees and Allowances Payable to General Medical Practitioners in England and Wales (The Red Book), DHSS (Welsh Office), National Health Service, General Medical Services, HMSO

Using the Laboratory (DHSS), HMSO

Which Benefit?, (DHSS), HMSO

Telephone numbers

Alcoholics Anonymous ....

Ambulance ....

BMA ....

Chemists ....

Chiropodist ....

Citizens Advice Bureau ....

Community Physician ....

Coroner..

Defence Society ....

Dentists...

DHSS Local Office ....

District Health Authority ....

District Nurse ....

Education Welfare Officer ....

Family and Child Guidance ....

Family Practitioner Committee ....

GMC ....

Health Visitors ....

Home Help Co-ordinator ....

Hospitals..

Telephone numbers

Marriage Guidance ....

Meals on Wheels ....

Midwives...

Nursing Officer ....

Occupational Therapist ....

Partners..

Physiotherapists ....

Police ....

Poisons Information Service..

Probation Service ....

Red Cross ....

RCGP..

RSPCA ....

Samaritans ....

Social Workers..

Social Worker Emergency No. ....

Surgeries/Health Centres...

Taxis ....

Undertakers ....

VD Clinic..

Voluntary Agencies ....

Index

Page references in *italic* type refer to charts, diagrams and tables.

Index

Index